STAY IN MEDICINE

HOW PHYSICIANS CAN MOVE PAST BURNOUT AND REGAIN CONTROL

**JANET CRUZ M.D.
AND LEE M.J. ELIAS**

Save Yourself,
Save Your Patients,
Save Medicine

Stay in Medicine
How Physicians Can Move Past Burnout and Regain Control
Janet Cruz M.D. and Lee M.J. Elias © 2021

All rights reserved. Use of any part of this publication, whether reproduced, transmitted in any form or by any means, electronic, mechanical, photocopying, recording, or otherwise, or stored in a retrieval system, without the prior consent of the publisher, is an infringement of copyright law and is forbidden.

While the publisher and author have used their best efforts in preparing this book, they make no representations or warranties with respect to the accuracy or completeness of this book and specifically disclaim any implied warranties of merchantability or fitness for a particular purpose. No warranty may be created or extended by sales representatives or written sales materials. Neither the publisher nor the author shall be liable for any loss of profit or any other commercial damages, including but not limited to special, incidental, consequential, or other damages. The stories and interviews in this book are true although the names and identifiable information may have been changed to maintain confidentiality.

The publisher and author shall have neither liability nor responsibility to any person or entity with respect to loss, damage, or injury caused or alleged to be caused directly or indirectly by the information contained in this book. The information presented herein is in no way intended as a substitute for counseling or other professional guidance.

The views expressed in this book are those of the authors and do not reflect the official policy or position of the U.S. Air Force, Department of Defense, or the U.S. government.

Cover Design Credit: Mirko Pohle
Photo Credit: Ann Marie Casey | amcphotostudios.com
Interior Design by Fusion Creative Works, FusionCW.com
Editorial Team: Megan Terry, Jennifer Regner, and Maryanna Young

Hardcover ISBN: 978-1-61206-229-7
Softcover ISBN: 978-1-61206-230-3
eBook ISBN: 978-1-61206-231-0

For more information, visit StayInMedicine.com

To purchase this book for your healthcare team or healthcare system, contact Aloha Publishing at alohapublishing@gmail.com or visit AlohaPublishing.com

Published by

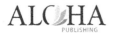

Printed in the United States of America

Dedications

FROM JANET:

To the village that helped me get into medicine, and to the village I would like to create to keep us in medicine.

To my husband, who has my pulse and pushes me to change the world.

To my mother, who showed me that coming from simple means is an advantage, and who has guided me to become the compassionate, feisty physician I am today.

To my family, the initial village that allowed me to stand on their shoulders so that I could have a different view.

To my children, Daddy and I have written an entire book together and there are still not enough words for us to convey how much we love you.

To my colleagues in medicine for the conversations that started at the end of shifts, late at night, or on weekends when we were "off duty," and who showed me how we need to continue to be advocates for our patients.

To you, the reader. Let's make a better world together.

FROM LEE:

For my wife, Janet. You wear many hats as a mother, wife, daughter, sister, family member, and friend.

Watching you pursue your dream of becoming a doctor has been humbling and frustrating, but above all it has been a blessing. I love you.

Contents

What If . . .	9
Chapter 1: Set Boundaries to Prevent Burnout	17
Chapter 2: Recover Time and Control	31
Chapter 3: Reduce Time-Killers	45
Chapter 4: Refocus on Patient Relationships	75
Chapter 5: Find Connection to Reframe Physician Isolation	95
Chapter 6: Create a Team Culture	113
Chapter 7: Become a Physician Leader	135
Change Can Start With You	145
References	149
Acknowledgments	155
About the Authors	159
Join Our Community	165

What If . . .

. . . THERE WERE NO DOCTORS?

Imagine for a moment that in the near future, you suddenly wake up with severe abdominal pain. You turn to your spouse, friend, or partner and ask for some water, hoping that will settle it. As the pain gets worse, you break into a sweat—nausea takes over and the pain becomes blinding. You can't get comfortable. You forget your plans and realize you can't take much more of this. Something is really wrong. What could it be? Your appendix? IBD? Just a bad burrito?

No matter what it is, it's time to see a doctor. Except . . . doctors are now hard to find.

In this future world, healthcare has changed. At the turn of the century, signs of the problem started to appear. Doctors had begun to leave medicine. Treating it like most ailments, the healthcare community trucked along, ignoring the obvious need for change. As the years progressed, more and more physicians left the profession. Word started getting out that doctors were leaving, and even medical school applications started to drop off. More and more college students realized that a career in medicine was too demanding and costly, with little reward or control. They realized that to be a doctor was to lead a lonely life of sacrifice.

In this future, some practicing physicians really tried to hold on. They did everything they could to remind each other of what they were supposed to stand for. But as hard as those physicians tried, it was too little, too late. As a result, medical schools across the country are competing for lower and lower enrollments. Intelligent, knowledgeable young people looking for a career realize that becoming a physician isn't worth the debt and pain.

Now at the mid-century mark, a true physician is hard to find and only those willing to spend exorbitant amounts of money have access.

Still in pain and desperate, you go to an urgent care where there is no physician in the building. You are evaluated, warned that it is more than a bad burrito, and instructed to follow up with "a doctor." But you don't have one and you don't know where to start looking.

You start to panic—what if this is serious? What if you can't get the care you need? It's looking like you might require surgery—and because of the doctor shortage, the wait times for that are weeks at best, and survival rates are continually decreasing.

WHAT IF IT'S NOT TOO LATE TO DO SOMETHING?

Okay, this story is getting dark. It sounds scary, doesn't it? But is this scenario that farfetched? In a country that spends more money per capita in the healthcare system than any other in the world (McCarthy, 2019), we have glaring and expanding gaps in our medical system. A scenario not too different from the nightmare I just described plays out across many states and U.S. territories today.

Even having insurance does not guarantee access to a physician. Medical care is more expensive than it's ever been. In many rural areas, patients are subjected to long wait times and long drives with no guarantee of seeing a physician. Patients in urban areas with numerous health systems are not exempt from this either. There may

WHAT IF . . .

be plenty of physicians and medical facilities, but what happens when the hospital system won't take your insurance?

In some countries, the idea of losing access to healthcare as a result of changing jobs is foreign, but in the U.S., this is commonplace. Our current system has uneven distribution of physicians in the midst of an underlying physician shortage. The population has increasingly incomplete medical coverage.

These trends are not new. Is this the system we want?

For those who may believe the nightmare "no doctors" scenario will never happen, let's not ignore some sobering statistics. A 2018 survey by the Physicians Foundation found that 46 percent of doctors surveyed planned to change career paths. Twelve percent want a job where they don't have to deal with patients (Pipes, 2018). For many physicians, medicine is not what we envisioned . . . not what we signed up for. At least half of physicians would not recommend healthcare as a profession to others.

TAKE A LOOK AROUND *TODAY*

Physicians and healthcare systems are at a precipice right now. It's time we have a serious conversation about where we want to go together. If we don't know where we are going, we will never get there.

How do we figure out where to go? It starts with asking great questions. Great questions demand great answers. So let me ask the first question that's on all of our minds:

Will staying in the medical field fulfill my soul and give me purpose?

That question breeds other questions: Is it time to walk away, or should I stay and strive to change the field? Is the sacrifice, dehumanization, and abuse we experience every day worth holding onto? What am I holding onto anymore?

STAY IN MEDICINE

I know I am not alone with these sentiments. Over the last five years, I've seen many physicians look for alternative careers to exit the complicated life medicine has become.

We are seeing a trend. Physicians are leaving medicine. We are tired, overworked, undervalued, and dissatisfied—and the most sacred relationships we hold, the ones with our patients, are slipping from our hands.

So what if physicians leave? There will be more to replace the ones leaving, right? Wrong again. How many of your friends or family are waiting longer to see a doctor? Or, they can no longer see their doctor because their insurance will no longer cover their visits. How many times were you forced to go to another hospital because your choice of doctor wasn't in your network?

Can you imagine a world where you couldn't get the care you needed in the United States? A world where you couldn't see a doctor? It seems so farfetched, but it is already starting. Private practices are struggling to survive due to the decreasing reimbursement rates from insurance companies and takeovers by large hospital systems. Advance practice practitioners (APPs) are on the rise as physician numbers decline.

It's time to fix our present so we can fortify our future.

WHERE CAN WE START?

While there are systemic issues we must ultimately address, I believe physicians have more power than they realize. You can make a difference in your daily work environment through your own actions with your team.

We have teams to help us and a dedicated medical community that is well aware of the issues we face. We must take more active leadership roles for our teams and redistribute tasks that don't require a physician's knowledge to others on the team. We need to

WHAT IF . . .

get help from IT to streamline our use of EMR and eliminate the administrative burdens of caring for patients.

The day-to-day reality for employed physicians is pretty much a guaranteed recipe for burnout. We must take a step back and look at what we can do to reduce the chaos in our own clinics.

For over a decade, discussions on issues like burnout have accelerated, and for good reason. By medical standards, we should be closer to a cure, based on the amount of time and effort spent. So why is this still an issue? Why are physicians leaving after committing so much time to learning a once highly sought-after profession? With primary care and specialty shortages, especially in underserved areas, we as a society cannot afford to let this situation continue.

The purpose of this book is not to "solve" these issues. I simply want to begin the conversations that need to take place.

Here's what we need to do:

- Regain control of our livelihood.
- Reignite our collective passion for practicing medicine.
- Ultimately, disrupt the system that is driving physicians out of medicine so we can once again practice medicine the way we want to.

Agree with me? Good. Don't agree with me? Great! Let's get a conversation started.

LET'S START THE CONVERSATION

Together, we can go beyond just discussing the problems and start taking action. I am Dr. Janet Cruz and along with my husband and co-author, Lee Elias, we are on a mission to help physicians restructure their lives. We want to help you deal with the big challenges in healthcare to create a lifestyle you can live with and even thrive in. We want to help you and those around you form a team you can be proud of. I am in the trenches, so I know what the struggles are.

My introduction to medicine was unique. Along with my siblings, I served as my parents' personal translators during medical appointments because, being from Puerto Rico, they didn't speak English. I became an advocate for my parents. Those interactions fueled me, and I felt a calling to primary care. I wanted to provide services to patients who were just like my parents.

I joined the military and was able to finance my medical school studies through the Air Force Health Careers Scholarship Program. My medical school experience was like most other medical students'—a cycle of physical and mental endurance. Similar to over 40 percent of medical students, I'd already begun to feel the exhaustion of my field (Davenport, 2018).

My journey with the Air Force was invaluable but also one of the most challenging experiences I have ever endured. I lived in multiple states and countries and learned to see medicine through a different lens than traditional medical training gives most physicians. Officer training gave me a unique perspective on my leadership role within medicine. I was expected to be an officer first, before being a physician. It was in the Air Force where my struggle with burnout really began.

I have continued to struggle with burnout throughout my career. Practicing medicine is where I want to be, so I made the decision that something needed to change.

I could not resign myself to a life where I dreaded going to work.

I began to search for ways to reinvigorate my passion for medicine and to help my colleagues who also were facing burnout.

WHAT IF . . .

What started as a project to keep myself in medicine evolved into something bigger, and you're reading this book as a result. The reasons I went into medicine are the same reasons that keep me from leaving.

In this book, I will outline the current climate that leads to burnout in physicians and other healthcare providers, as well as other issues facing our profession. I will share the solutions I have devised to help each of us handle burnout in our own lives—to start making a difference now. I'll also share my perspective on issues that need change on a larger scale.

Here are a few of the big things happening in U.S. medicine today. These demonstrate how we need larger change:

- Healthcare is overpriced, for many reasons. It's not the cost of services—it's the cost of everything else. It's difficult to track the source of the expenses.

- The healthcare environment has become difficult for physicians because they can't negotiate with insurance companies. Reimbursements from insurance are only getting smaller. Patients are billed more and physicians make less. Patients are paying higher premiums as well as higher copays. Why, and what is the product they are receiving?

- Forces (insurance companies and pharmaceutical companies) are lobbying to keep healthcare costs high. This is happening at least partly in opposition to recent (2018-2020) proposed bills designed to reduce pharmaceutical and healthcare costs.

- More physicians are employed than ever before, instead of being in charge of their own clinics. Because of this, they often don't even know what the patient is charged.

STAY IN MEDICINE

- Expectations for physicians have grown, although there is no more time in the day. The growing list of tasks and requirements lead to longer and more exhausting work hours.

- Increasing cost-saving measures by insurance companies create barriers to effective and timely care of patients. At the same time, those measures increase the administrative burdens on physicians.

- Many physicians are leaving medicine due to burnout.

- Physicians are some of the most resilient of professionals, yet they have one of the highest suicide rates.

Many people know about the burnout epidemic in medicine, and in some ways, it has been the canary in the coal mine. Burnout is shedding light on what really ails the medical system.

Let's take that a step further and redirect the conversation toward solutions. Let's keep ourselves and those who have contributed to creating this situation accountable as we connect.

1

Set Boundaries to Prevent Burnout

> **Problem:** Physicians experience overwhelming burnout.
>
> **What you control:** How you identify and handle your own burnout and how you support your colleagues who are experiencing burnout.
>
> **Action items:** Define your personal mission and what gets in the way of that mission to begin seeking solutions . . . and read this book.

We all have a story regarding our burnout.

Burnout stories in medicine are common. They are also diverse—each physician's burnout story has its own background and circumstances. There is a shared feeling among these stories, not of regret, but of resolve. While we may at times feel frustrated, exhausted, or completely lost, we remember the passion that inspired us to get into this field.

Finding that passion again is part of the key to moving forward.

Throughout this book, I will share some of my own stories. I'm doing this for two reasons: to give context and tangibility to what

I am trying to discuss and to encourage you to share your stories as well. I want everyone to realize that while no two stories are the same, we all experience similar issues. You are not alone, and through sharing these stories we can find strength.

Conversations in the office can help to diffuse frustration, but that doesn't change what's happening or why. Information about how the healthcare system fails to provide is presented in medical journals that patients rarely see. The conversation needs to expand to include patients—we need to create transparency and visibility for all who are impacted.

As healthcare providers, we see situations on a daily basis that create rifts between us and our patients. Patients feel it personally. They often feel dissatisfied with their interactions within the healthcare system.

There is a dire need to elevate the discussions we have in our clinics to a larger platform like social media. This would help us to discuss the current healthcare climate and allow patients to engage with us.

Ultimately, patients need to become active partners and participants if we want to fix the system.

BATTLING A CULTURE OF BURNOUT

Within a year of residency training as a young Air Force captain, I hit the ground running. Soon, I learned I wasn't prepared for a life in medicine. It was not the lack of medical training that made things difficult. It was a lack of training in everything else that is now required to successfully work in medicine.

SET BOUNDARIES TO PREVENT BURNOUT

After a couple months of working on my own, I felt helpless, frayed, and worn. At one point, I talked to a friend who was not in the medical field and rattled off all the things wrong with my job.

Her solution for me was this: "Just quit."

I nearly exploded with anger. "Just quit? And do what, exactly?"

I'd spent the better part of my youth trying to get here—countless hours studying, missing family events and social gatherings. I ate, breathed, and lived medicine, and I loved it for a time. In medical school, I enjoyed talking to patients, helping them identify their problems, providing education, and learning from them.

But once I finished medical school, the day-to-day was impossible to escape. I was buried in tasks and the stress plagued my home life. I couldn't stop thinking about the tasks I missed during the day. How could I call everyone back and address all the lab results in time?

I slowly came to resent my career choice and the patients I served. There was even a time when the thought of walking into my clinic made me nauseous. What's even more disturbing is my story echoes the feelings of so many other physicians. Where did things go wrong?

The saddest thing to me was that I literally couldn't quit. At the time, I was an active duty military physician. Quitting is not an option when you belong to the government.

I slowly became disillusioned with medicine. I felt my career was spiraling out of control. This was not what I signed up for. How much of my time was actually spent problem-solving for patients? Almost none. Throughout the day, I would make lists of conditions I wanted to look up and new treatment plans or medical articles I wanted to read. Instead, I ended up tackling lists of medication refill requests, prior authorization forms, work and school excuse notes, and modifications for work exemptions. Add to that the 20-plus patients I saw on most days. By the time I was done, I had no time left to think about medicine.

My work bled into my home life until there was no delineation. The tasks were endless and the demand to see more patients only increased. The slogan "Patients need more access" was repeated during numerous meetings, yet the workforce shrank due to deployments or temporary duty assignments.

I couldn't keep up with everything demanded of me. I was a military officer, a leader, a supervisor, and a physician. And for my patients, care was served on a platter of apologies. "I'm sorry for being late." "I'm sorry it took me a couple days to call you back." I was just sorry. I was taking responsibility for system failures.

I felt like I held rice in my hand, with more grains slipping between my fingers the tighter I gripped. I had no idea how to handle it all. It soon was apparent that neither did my colleagues.

I did what most of my colleagues did—got up earlier, stayed at work later, and worked harder. Initially, I listened to my older colleagues. They said the first year out of training was an adjustment and tough for everyone.

I went to work at 5 a.m. routinely and didn't leave until 7 or 8 p.m. I skipped lunch and bathroom breaks in an attempt to "catch up." But it soon became clear it wasn't my inexperience or work ethic dragging me down. The work didn't get any easier. I became numb. I cheered when patients didn't show for appointments. I resented them when they were late or when they asked questions not related to the reason for their visit.

That was when I knew there was a problem, and my first crisis began.

How was I going to make a 20-plus-year career out of this?
I was two years in and losing it.

SET BOUNDARIES TO PREVENT BURNOUT

I tried all the "tricks" recommended by senior colleagues. I read all the literature I could find on physician burnout, listened to motivational speakers, and infused my office with essential oils. And while these efforts helped some, the piles of work didn't go anywhere.

It didn't matter how much I meditated or how many positivity quotes I recited. I started my mornings, like every other physician, with a long task list I knew I would never get through. This list was on top of my appointments for the day that I knew would generate more work. The patients became the barrier keeping me from my family.

This routine was and still is a known culture in medicine, an accepted way of life. The life of a doctor is always busy. My colleagues and I took turns carrying each other through the burnout. We checked in with each other. We plowed through our patient appointments and reviewed labs and radiologic studies in any spare second we had. We piled on meetings and administrative tasks in place of eating, bathroom breaks, exercise, and time spent with family.

When I couldn't take it anymore, a colleague stepped in and sent me home. He stayed late and made a dent in my work, to give me just a little reprieve. And when he was in the same place of burnout, I returned the favor.

However, sharing or trading tasks with other physicians is not a solution. It is not sustainable.

I was a shell of myself when I came home to my husband, with nothing left to offer. I was exhausted after talking all day and rushing through tasks. I had no control over my world. That is what burnout looks like. Lee calls those times "the dark days." It is a reality that many of my colleagues are living today.

I wish I could say the camaraderie of my colleagues was enough, but it wasn't. During my first year as an attending, we lost a provider after he suffered a heart attack and then was hospitalized again for suicidal ideation. He was forced to leave his position as a military physician. To add insult to injury, my colleagues and I were not allowed to escort him to another base because we were told we couldn't leave patient care.

Other colleagues of mine left primary care too and took administrative jobs. How many of the six colleagues I started out with actually stayed in primary care? Just me. One out seven. That is the cost of burnout.

Nationally, we lose approximately 400 providers a year, according to a 10-year literature review presented by the American Psychiatry Association in 2018 (Anderson, 2018; Farmer, 2018). With all the studies that show the effects of physician burnout, what are we doing as a system to rectify the situation? How are we holding healthcare systems and ourselves accountable?

In our current healthcare climate, burnout is treated as an individual problem rather than a systemic one. Many articles are written about meditation, personality analysis of physicians, and other methods to handle burnout. These are all focused on how physicians can reform themselves to combat burnout. It is framed as a problem within each of us.

In my seven years as an attending, I completed at least five mandatory computer-based trainings on physician burnout—to be done on my own time. Did my nurses, medical technicians, administrators, or health insurance providers have to take these trainings? Of course not. This speaks volumes about how we as a system view this problem.

I cannot begin to say how deflating it is to be told, "You have to complete this training by the end of the week," when you have no dedicated time to do so. I heard one of my nurse colleagues ask our administrator if she needed to complete the mandatory training as well. The reply was, "No, this is mandatory for the docs. You don't have to worry about that training."

SET BOUNDARIES TO PREVENT BURNOUT

How effective do you think that computer-based training on physician burnout was for me, as I plowed through it at home in place of eating with my family?

I always knew being a physician would take me away from my family, but I had assumed it would be in order to take call and answer medical questions. It is not.

BURNOUT IS SYSTEMIC

I believe physician burnout is a symptom of a larger systemic issue. It is a culmination of how medicine has changed throughout the years, leaving patients and physicians alike feeling hopeless, powerless, and unfulfilled. Where did things go wrong?

> *Where and when did a profession of service turn into a profession of servitude?*

In this book, I illustrate the underlying causes of burnout so that, together, we can find real solutions to bring about change. This is absolutely critical for a system that no longer functions for either the people providing the service or those receiving it. Only from that point can we begin tackling the other issues facing the medical community.

While you may already be familiar with burnout, each one of us experiences it differently. It's important that we approach it with a similar understanding.

WHAT DOES BURNOUT LOOK LIKE?

Some people say burnout is a manifestation of depression. And while depression may contribute to burnout and vice versa, they are not the same thing. But similar to depression, burnout will start to invade all aspects of your life.

Typical signs of burnout include the following:

- Feelings of defeat and/or helplessness
- A sense of self-doubt and failure
- Despondency and feelings of isolation
- Loss of motivation
- Inability to focus or complete tasks
- Difficulty finding satisfaction or a sense of accomplishment at work
- A persistent negative outlook

Burnout has a great impact on the quality of care that is delivered to patients. Ultimately, it affects our safety as providers and the safety of our patients.

WHAT ARE THE LONG-TERM COSTS OF BURNOUT?

The current healthcare environment that leads to burnout is not a personal or individual problem. It is systemic, yet it is not treated as such. We know that the amount of face-to-face time between a physician and a patient has decreased from 25 percent to 17 percent of a physician's time, according to reports from the American Council of Science and Health (Kane, 2019).

We don't need statistics to tell us this information. I have seen it and felt it. I have spent more time each day documenting my encounters with patients than actually talking to them.

We work in a system that prides itself on data collection and analysis, but how often do we collect data in our own clinics? Do we use this data to help guide our decisions?

SET BOUNDARIES TO PREVENT BURNOUT

According to the 2019 Medscape National Physician Burnout, Depression and Suicide Report surveying nearly 15,000 physicians, approximately 44 percent are burned out (Kane, 2019). As a result, 40 percent are more likely to work part time or leave clinical medicine altogether. According to recent data published by the AAMC (Association of American Medical Colleges), a shortage of nearly 122,000 physicians is predicted by 2032, not including the loss of physicians currently leaving medicine due to burnout (Spector, 2018).

In the current environment, when there is already a physician shortage, we can't afford to lose more physicians. For primary care, the cost of replacing a physician is two to three times the physician's annual salary. And beyond the cost of hiring, the shortage of physicians affects patient care. It limits physician availability and decreases quality of care due to burnout.

What's even more shocking is medical students are already burned out by the time they get through medical school.

Physicians have an increased risk of death due to their profession. It is estimated that 400 medical students and physicians commit suicide annually in the U.S. The suicide rate is up to 3.8 times higher for male physicians and 4.5 times higher for female physicians compared to the general population (Farmer, 2018).

The data has been published in high-quality medical journals and broadcast in mainstream media. Attempts to change the system are often thwarted by the bottom dollar—the costs outweigh the benefits in the eyes of the decision-makers.

More importantly, the quality of patient care is decreasing. Data shows increasing distrust in the medical system, increasing medical errors, and increasing delays in care due to the fragmented system (Khullar, 2018).

STAY IN MEDICINE

The long-term costs of burnout are high for both physicians and patients.

ADDRESSING BURNOUT ON AN INDIVIDUAL BASIS

In my journey to combat my personal struggles with burnout, I saw the wreckage the medical field has experienced. The solutions that have been offered to me were like Band-Aids—they did nothing to address the largest contributors to the hostile environment of the healthcare system: lack of connection, lack of relationships, and lack of ethics.

I recognize that there are aspects of the path to becoming a physician that contribute to burnout. After all, it takes a vast amount of organization, delayed gratification, and general grit to get through the demands of undergraduate and medical school. The problem is the long hours and huge lists of tasks don't end with completing residency. That's just the beginning.

It isn't medicine that is driving physicians out—it is the system we are forced to work with in our profession.

THE FIVE LOSSES

I've identified the aspects of my job as a physician that have led to my burnout. I refer to these as the five losses:

- Loss of control
- Loss of time
- Loss of relationships
- Loss of connection
- Loss of team

I've changed my approach to issues that previously resulted in my burnout. I now carve out time in the day to intentionally analyze my clinic and environment. When I am thinking about a problem, I begin by asking myself a simple question:

Is this something I can control?

In answering this question, I find clarity. I cannot control everything, and I cannot do my job alone.

> ***If I am staying in medicine, I have to be part of the force that changes it for the better.***

Throughout this book, you'll see outlines of the most common culprits of the toxic and exhausting environment in the medical field. You'll also see a structure I've identified for addressing the problems within the healthcare system. Using these solutions, we can create the momentum needed to change the system, starting with your day-to-day experience.

We will go through the strategies I used to help with the five losses. You will find a systematic approach to analyzing your environment and surrounding yourself with the right people to help implement change. As professionals, we can lift up and encourage each other. This is something well within our control as individuals.

If you're burned out like I was, let's take a step forward together.

TAKE 10

Take 10 minutes to answer the following questions:

1. What is your mission? Do your team members or organization share the same mission?

2. What are your daily obligations?

3. Are you able to complete your daily obligations and if not, what tasks are you unable to complete?

4. If you answered no to question 3, why are you unable to complete those tasks?

5. If you are interrupted during the day by issues/tasks that are unaccounted for in your schedule and workload, what are they?

Write your answers on a piece of paper and keep it somewhere you will remember or use it as a bookmark as you read this book.

SET BOUNDARIES TO PREVENT BURNOUT

CHAPTER 1 WRAP-UP

Your medical training has conditioned you to expect work overload and long days. This pattern is not sustainable, year after year. As an attending, there's a point where you need to set boundaries on how much work you must do in a day. This is critical in order to preserve your ability to effectively and sustainably practice medicine. It may require a new mindset about the tasks on your list, and a new set of decision-making skills—how to work with your team to spread the workload more evenly and provide the best patient care possible. The cause of burnout may be systemic, but the first steps toward lightening your load can be accomplished by you with a new perspective.

Join the conversation at
StayInMedicine.com

2

Recover Time and Control

> **Problem:** Physicians feel they have little control over their schedule, their lives, or the healthcare system.
>
> **What you control:** Your decisions, actions, and things in your direct environment.
>
> **Action items:** Identify what you do and do not control and focus only on what you control.

To practice medicine effectively, we need to gain control over ourselves and our time. We simply cannot provide stability and care to others if we don't provide it to ourselves first—you cannot give someone something you don't have.

To achieve this, we must put hard limits in place in order to be better at our jobs. We need to learn to rely on others and a team, instead of the knee-jerk response of taking on more and more individual responsibilities and tasks. That isn't realistic or sustainable. We allow and expect our patients to be human—not robots—and we can allow ourselves the same liberty.

Let's start by talking about the obvious:

STAY IN MEDICINE

Time is finite and no one can control everything.

In medicine, it often feels like these rules don't apply. We are expected to find time that doesn't exist and control the uncontrollable. I hear "Just make time!" over and over again. It can't be done. Making time for anything requires sacrificing something else. But the solution is not simply to throw in the towel. Instead, let's keep time and control in the forefront of what we do.

We must treat the time we have as a valuable resource. The attitude that says, "Just take care of it," or "It just has to get done," has cost those serving in medicine greatly.

In reality, the responsibility for patient care is placed mostly on the physician. Based on current guidance, an individual physician does not have enough time in the day to properly address the preventative measures recommended for your patients. In spite of that, the expectation that you will do all those things hasn't changed.

For example, in 2003, the American Journal of Public Health published a study regarding how long it would take a primary care physician to complete all the preventative measures recommended by the U.S. Preventive Services Task Force (USPSTF). The USPSTF is a governance body that generates guidelines based on existing medical literature and consensus on what will keep a population healthy. This study reported that, as a primary care physician, you would need 7.4 hours per working day (1773 hours of a physician's annual time) to meet the preventive care needs of your patients, if you have 2,500 patients in your practice (Yarnall et al., 2003).

After working in various clinics in different parts of the country, I can tell you it is impossible to meet those goals without help. I would have to spend almost all day providing just this service. In

RECOVER TIME AND CONTROL

real life, I see three to four wellness visits a day, and a patient typically gets 30 minutes to talk about preventative measures.

How we meet these goals is a big factor in how our practices are paid. This study outlines the expectations without true accountability of the time commitment needed to fulfill these goals.

Furthermore, there is a culture in medicine that assigns responsibility to a single person. In one incident, a patient was discharged from the hospital. An intern meticulously wrote all the patient's medications down in the discharge summary. The discharge summary and the medications were supposed to be delivered to the patient before they left the hospital. But the nurse never printed out the discharge summary and did not review it with the patient. The physician was unaware of the error until a couple of weeks later, when the patient returned to the ER for the exact same condition.

Cases like these are examined in morbidity and mortality reviews, which don't incorporate all the other elements required to take care of the patient. In this case, the blame fell on the intern for not checking to make sure the patient received their medications. Where is the accountability of other team members in addition to ourselves? What about the nurse who didn't follow the physician's orders?

You may think this is as an isolated incident. Trust me, it is not. The number of "workarounds" created on the backs of physicians to prevent the recurrence of a similar event prevents these issues from rising to the surface.

In the current system, if something doesn't get done, the physician has to add that task to their list—and your time is allocated to another task that doesn't need your level of expertise.

You cannot control everything in your environment. We know this but rarely acknowledge it. It is easy to get overwhelmed. Pressure comes in all forms, but how much of the pressure you feel is self-imposed? How often do you feel like a failure when you are unable to keep up with the unrealistic demands on your time? The expectation that you must take on administrative tasks in addition to practicing medicine are not only unrealistic, they are making chaos out of the day-to-day workload.

We read about burnout in the medical journals and we see it in each other's faces. We experience it in the time we spend after hours, completing tasks or creating workarounds for a system that is broken and bureaucratic. It's easy to feel helpless beneath the pressure.

THE LOSS OF CONTROL

As physicians, it seems we don't have much control over our day-to-day lives. The tasks are insurmountable and sometimes we're treated more like machines than people. When I began writing this book, I initially felt like a fraud. How could I advise others to change the system when I felt burned out too? My daily life felt out of control.

For the majority of jobs in the U.S., there are regulations on how long you can work. The legal limit is typically 80 hours a week. In medicine, that limit only applies during your training years. Once you're done being a resident, there are no hour restrictions.

When I was a new Air Force physician, I would see patients in the clinic during the day and go to the hospital in the middle of the night to do my admissions. No matter how late I worked, I had to wake up for work the next day.

How many times have you heard stories of a physician who had the stomach bug and came to work because no one could cover their shift? They got an IV of fluids and medications prior to their shift to prevent vomiting, and they were expected to work. This happens all the time.

In residency, you're given a list of tasks to do and told to just get it done—whatever it takes. Residency was one of my biggest challenges. It wasn't because of the immense amount of learning or the long hours. I loved medicine—seeing new cases and hearing amazing stories from my patients. I knew it would be a lot to handle, but I felt the pressure to manage it and constantly told myself, "Just put your head down and get to work." And I went to one of the most supportive, mindful residency programs.

At that time, I was so busy and immersed in my role as a physician that things began to fall through the cracks. The water service to my house was shut off because I forgot to pay the bill. I was always rushing to get to work or to finish work.

I wish I could say I had an epiphany when the water was shut off to get me to take care of myself. But the same kind of incident happened again and again in other aspects of my life.

It wasn't until I was 36 weeks pregnant with my son, Logan, one year after completing my residency, that the message to take care of myself finally stuck. I was still seeing a full schedule of patients and staying at the office until 6:30 p.m.—documenting the work of the day and tackling the endless labs and patient phone messages.

Lee called and said, "Janet, what are you doing? You're about to have a baby. Get out of the office already."

I'm not saying pregnant women aren't capable of working long days, because we are. The hours I was pulling were beyond ridiculous, pregnant or not. I understood what Lee was trying to say. At that time, I woke up at 5 a.m. and went to work to accomplish administrative tasks before my first patient arrived. I worked through lunch, stayed in the office well past closing time to get everything done, and then picked up calls at night for internal medicine. It wasn't just me—we all did it. This is the norm for physicians, and this day was no different.

STAY IN MEDICINE

On the same night I got that call from my husband, I went into labor. I gave birth to my son 24 hours later, with Lee and my colleagues by my side.

I had been contracting all week and didn't even notice. I was lost in my job, keeping my head down, and determined to make a dent in my work. I needed to learn to identify my needs and take care of myself.

Stories like this are pervasive in the medical field: Failing to get your own physical because there just isn't any time. Coming to work sick with a cold. Why? Because of the overwhelming guilt that you will have to reschedule 20-25 patients who are "sicker" than you and probably have waited months to see you.

That particular day, I was forced to slow down because I was in labor. That was when I began to analyze what I was doing. I was constantly stressed, my mind cluttered with things I could not control.

In waking up to the fact that I needed to take care of myself, I had to acknowledge a couple of things I wasn't doing that could be part of the solution:

1. I needed to start living in the now.
2. I needed to learn what I could actually control.

In those two simple principles, I found clarity.

Start with identifying what you actually can control. You cannot control every element of your environment, but you can recognize shortcomings. You can focus on making changes to things you do have control over and empower others to do the same.

In order to gain control over your life, I would like to introduce two guiding principles: the **circle of control** and **living in the now**.

RECOVER TIME AND CONTROL

CIRCLE OF CONTROL

Lee, who constantly works with various types of teams, is always telling me, "Only focus on the things in your life you can control." Every time he says that I want to roll my eyes. The thought that pops into my mind is, *If I don't have control over this, it's no different from everything else. I feel out of control most of the time.* Like most things in marriage, we were both right and we were both wrong.

He was right that focusing on what you can control individually allows you to be more effective in your daily life. However, as an individual, there are limits to what you can control. That's why you need a team. As a team, the scope of control is much wider and systemic challenges can be conquered more easily.

When we say, "Focus on what you can control," we are referring to what you can actually control in the moment. That is, what you can attack right now to help you get to the next moment. If each person on your team takes this approach, it will help achieve the common goal as a group. Here are some suggestions:

Build in time for yourself. Make time to eat, time to use the restroom, time to call your loved ones, time if you are a mother to breast-pump, or time to just breathe. Then protect that time. These are basic necessities. Don't ignore them. You are in control of your behavior and your actions. Creating time for yourself is one of them. You can choose to build this into your day, just like a patient appointment. This needs to happen.

Set boundaries. Educate your team on how to take care of situations in your absence. To not do so is setting them up to fail. Resentment builds up when you are trying to get your work done and are constantly interrupted by your staff. Or, when you finally sit down to eat only to have a staff member tell you a patient showed up early and wants to be seen now.

STAY IN MEDICINE

Learn how to say no. As a physician, everyone wants your time. Learning to say no doesn't mean you have to automatically reject projects or turn away staff when they have questions for you, but you don't have to commit to everything.

Unclutter your mind. Take the time to unclutter your thoughts. Yes, this means practicing mindfulness. It does not necessarily mean picking up yoga or knitting—unless you want to. It is easy for your mind to wander into tomorrow, but it takes you away from what you are doing now. You control your thoughts.

I do not want to oversimplify this process. It is difficult and ongoing. After a three-year stay at a military base in England (my first job assignment), it was time for me to return home. About one month prior to my departure date, I received a phone call from the chief of medical staff from my receiving base. That was odd.

The colonel had tracked me down, internationally, while I was completing my shift in the ER. The conversation quickly brushed over formalities and got to the heart of the matter: The clinic I was about to lead had significant issues and he wanted to make sure I would hit the ground running. He gave me a long list of the ongoing issues and what he thought the clinic needed. At the end of the conversation, he expressed how delighted he was to have spoken to me and how he felt much calmer knowing I was coming.

That was a great interaction. However, I was left with my head spinning. What was I about to walk into? I felt overwhelmed and I hadn't even left England yet.

I had to step back and focus on the work I was doing. While it took a couple days to calm my anxiety, I had to stop living in the fears I had for my future. For a person who tries to prepare for everything, this was a change for me. It kept me from spiraling into the abyss. I chose not to focus on the unknown problems I would face. I focused on what I could do in the present moment. Panic would not help prepare me to make decisions effectively.

RECOVER TIME AND CONTROL

I had a pending overseas move and ER shifts I had to complete. I also had the advantage of knowing I was going to embark on a journey of rehabilitating a clinic. Lee and I made a checklist to help us focus on what we could control. I embraced my family and looked at resources that would help me analyze the clinic when I got there. Not only was this more manageable, it made me a more effective leader once I arrived.

LIVE IN THE NOW AND LIVE NOW

Reflect on the past, look to the future, but live in the present moment. If you take away anything from this book, let this make the cut!

In addition to understanding your circle of control, it is also important to live in the present moment. As humans, we perceive our reality through time. No matter what we do, the clock is ticking. We have no control over time—it marches on. If we perceive our existence through time, then our only reality is the present moment.

Have you ever been reading a book or a magazine only to realize that you don't remember anything from the past few pages? Your mind wandered somewhere else, and although you were reading the words, you were not retaining them. This is an example of not living in the now.

It's easy for anyone to get lost reliving the past or daydreaming about the future. You might lose focus by dwelling on a recent mistake or worrying about your financial future (among other things). While reflection and projection are healthy because you can learn from the past and set goals for the future, too much can hinder your ability to take action in the present. No amount of regret or money has ever bought a second of time.

Lee always compares my job to being a professional athlete. With the number of hours we put into perfecting our craft and into the job and the number of people who see us and remember us, he's not wrong. Athletes call living in the moment being "in the zone." If you've played or watched sports you might have experienced this as well: Everything seems to slow down and scoring (or however you earn points in the game you play) seems to come naturally. The focus is incredible and the results are undeniable. This is a practice we can adopt.

Living in the now can be difficult for physicians. We're planners. We tend to think days or months ahead. Because I work in academia, I may be doing research for a presentation at a conference six months from now. That's not what I mean by living in the now. What I mean is focusing on the task you're doing right now and not allowing other worries to distract you from it. Getting absorbed in your task helps release a lot of anxiety. It doesn't mean foregoing planning for the future. It means focusing more on what is in front of you right now.

You can look at the present in several ways. In some instances, it is quantified as the current month or week, or even the current day. During a workday in the medical field, the present becomes a second-by-second focus. This is why, no matter if a situation is good or bad, we should all strive to live in the now.

Focusing on the present creates a mental toughness that is important for high-pressure situations, which doctors face every day. When a person's health or life is on the line, every decision is vital. In these amplified situations, your ability to control your emotions is imperative. These are the moments when self-control and your ability to focus on what is in front of you will help you perform to your maximum potential.

The practice of focusing on the now is essential to finding balance both in life and in medicine. You cannot change your last action any more than you can predict the future. Staying mentally and emotionally focused in the moment will give you the best chance of succeeding.

RECOVER TIME AND CONTROL

We can also learn to set boundaries for ourselves. In medicine we often say, "Practice at the top of your scope." It is equally important to recognize our limitations and work within our capabilities.

Start by understanding how much work you're expected to complete in a day. What is actually possible? Eliminate factors that are unexpected and are not emergencies. Is the work you're supposed to do possible within the time that's been allocated?

The boundaries you set should exclude anything that is beyond the tasks allocated to the day. If they can't fit, something needs to come off your schedule before a new task is added on.

Set boundaries for yourself so you are not stretched beyond what you can provide on a physical or an emotional level. In addition to yourself, it's important to recognize when you or someone on your team is not focused on the current matter. Mentor your team on how to focus on the now and delegate responsibilities accordingly. Physicians should not be a bottleneck if a patient wants to get an appointment. Team members should take on tasks that don't require medical decisions.

Reflect on the past, look to the future, and live in the present moment.

> To reinforce these two concepts—focus on what you control and live in the present moment—each chapter in this book begins with three brief sentences that contain the **problem** we are discussing, **what you control** within your workspace, and the **action items** you can take in the present moment to find a solution.

TAKE 10

Take 10 minutes right now to create a list of items in your day-to-day that you control and items you don't. The list of items you control should be dramatically shorter. Post this list where you can see it daily and refer to it whenever you are stressed or are struggling to make a decision.

THINGS YOU CONTROL

_____
_____
_____
_____
_____
_____
_____
_____

THINGS YOU DON'T CONTROL

_____
_____
_____
_____
_____
_____
_____
_____

CHAPTER 2 WRAP-UP

Take a more strategic look at how you get through the day and try out a new perspective. Instead of assuming that all aspects of each patient's care are on your plate, look at each task with an eye for assigning anything you can to others on your team. By doing this, you *take control* of your schedule and your workload.

Practice deliberately evaluating each task to determine the skill set needed for that task, and engage your team to help them help you. Identifying what you *don't* have control over helps you see what you *do* have control over and can show you a way to change how that issue impacts you.

Join the conversation at
StayInMedicine.com

3

Reduce Time-Killers

Problem: There is too little time in the day to handle the number of tasks typically assigned to physicians. Plus, administrators don't understand the needs of patients or physicians and don't account for physician work outside the patient visit.

What you control: How you delegate/leverage tasks to team members and your efforts to implement processes to improve efficiency. You also control the dialogue you have with administration about unfair policies.

Action items: Delegate/leverage as much as possible and share your workload with your team. Communicate with administration and IT members about EMR system issues. Be transparent with your team, patients, and with administration about the struggles you face and how those get in the way of providing the best care to patients.

Time is your most valuable commodity. It's your measuring stick for your reality—we all perceive it one second at a time. It's a finite resource, so it's inherently valuable. How do you value your time?

Not just time at work but time for you, for your family, your team, and anything else you believe deserves your time.

We only have control over what we choose to do with the time we have. So how can we spend more time on the things we were trained for, and commit less time to tasks that do not serve us? How can we tap into everyone's time bank?

Do you spend your time doing things that only you can do?

After years of hearing the clichés "Use your time wisely," or "Use your team," I realized early in my career that I didn't have a good way of enacting these practices. Most of my colleagues didn't know how to truly use a team structure to work toward a common mission. Let's tackle some of the most common time-consumers and explore ways we can construct a team to best allocate time.

Over the course of this chapter, I will concentrate on the most common time-killers in a physician's day-to-day. Then, we'll outline the best strategies to collectively combat those issues by creating a team.

ADMINISTRATIVE CHALLENGES

Administrative challenges stem from systems that were developed to help but that now hinder physicians. We lose time doing paperwork instead of reading up on the patient. We lose time in meetings. *We never have enough time.* Administrative challenges overall are about time allocation. And for most of us, the two biggest problems are tasks outside the face-to-face patient encounter and the notorious electronic medical record (EMR) system. Let's start by tackling those first.

REDUCE TIME-KILLERS

Too Many Tasks Outside the Patient Visit

When you speak to patients and physicians, they complain about the same thing: there is just too much paperwork nowadays. For physicians, this is what really buries us. A colleague early in my military career described family medicine as "exsanguination by a million cuts." I replied, "Yep, paper cuts."

And now that most of the paperwork is electronic, the piles of paperwork are not as visible, but the result is the same or even worse. When you ask physicians what the most frustrating part of the day is, their answer isn't what you might expect. In 2016, this was clearly demonstrated in a study published in the *Annals of Internal Medicine*, which concluded that for every one hour of direct clinical face time, providers spent approximately two hours on EMR and desk work. They estimated that 27 percent of their total time was spent directly with patients and 49 percent with EMR and desk work. Some providers also reported one to two hours a day after hours required to complete EMR/desk work (Sinsky et al., 2016). This hasn't changed much as of today.

As a medical student, I knew I would have challenging patients—taking care of people is complicated. I knew I would have to tackle complex medical cases and the study of medicine would exceed the hours spent in the office. I knew being a physician was a calling and I would spend the rest of my life as both an expert and a perpetual student, since new and innovative ways of diagnosing and treating disease are constantly being developed. What I did not expect was finishing my charts at 10 p.m. in my pajamas after hurrying my kids to sleep . . . an event aptly called "pajama time" by many physicians.

There are so many tasks physicians are responsible for outside the face-to-face patient visit that it's impossible to complete everything within a "normal" workday. This hurried sprint results in rushed patient appointments, missed phone messages, delayed responses, and ultimately an increase in the risk for errors and harm to the patient.

On a typical day as an active-duty military physician, I would get to work at 6 or 6:30 a.m. and wouldn't leave until 6 or 7 p.m. I was almost never done seeing patients by the time lunch rolled around and there were inevitably at least one or two patients who walked in and needed to be seen as well. On occasion I'd have an unstable patient or an unexpected event during the day that would delay me further. Then I would try to catch up at night when the family was finally asleep.

I was never done. What I've outlined here doesn't even include the hours spent taking calls during nights and weekends for inpatient service or the time spent supervising other providers. When you look at the above, why would anyone go into medicine? Why would anyone stay?

During those days, I remember Lee asking, "How was your day?" and my response was always, "Busy."

I felt run down. I knew I was constantly hustling, but when I recalled my day, I couldn't easily account for anything other than my time with the patient. So for a day, I wrote down every interruption—any time I spent on completing a document or talking on the phone.

I was stunned. There were so many things that snuck into my day that I "just took care of" and no one accounted for them. No wonder I was wiped out at the end of the day. After several years, I realized completing all the tasks required to properly take care of patients is impossible without help.

What are the tasks you are expected to do? Where does your time go?

REDUCE TIME-KILLERS

Despite all the data demonstrating that people really don't multitask—we are only able to switch from one task to the other in an interrupted manner—we are faced with countless interruptions during the day. As a health system, we do not account for the amount of work required to take care of a patient.

Typically, staffing proportions are picked based on the number of face-to-face encounters alone. There is a misconception that this is the only factor that generates money. What about everything else we are responsible for during the day? What tasks or work is being missed or just not done due to lack of time?

Administrative tasks and non-face-to-face encounters need to be accounted for in determining staffing levels. In my experience, most medical organizations do not have the pulse on this.

So, in that simple exercise of tracking my time, I was able to see my time bank was depleted. But luckily for my clinic team, between all of us, we had loads of time.

What can you do as an individual, within your circle of control, to relieve some of the pressure of administrative tasks?

Here are four action items to get started:

1. Make a list of unplanned-for items and events that happen throughout the day.

You can't start to fix what is wrong if you can't show and articulate how all of these distractions lead to inefficiencies, delay in work completion, and ultimately poor service for patients. We all feel it, but we don't put it on paper.

2. What tasks are not accounted for that end up on your plate? Do these tasks have to be done by you? Can they be delegated to others?

Treat time as if it were tangible, like cash. Once you spend it, it's gone and any purchases after that are just debt. This is what commonly happens to us—we go through our clinics, collecting debt for the next day and find it hard to catch up. But as a collective, our spending power is a lot greater.

Do the tasks you complete require your expertise and training as a physician? If not, those tasks need to be delegated to others.

3. Identify and define the roles and responsibilities of everyone on your team. Who has time in their bank?

In my experience in several clinic and hospital settings, most team members don't know the scope of their jobs. Worse yet, their teammates and colleagues don't know the scope of each other's jobs. So how can we all practice to the top of our ability if we don't even know what our jobs entail? Physicians waste a lot of time trying to figure out who is responsible for doing particular tasks. And there is nothing more frustrating when we are hustling than seeing a team member taking their fifth break or casually conversing with a colleague. We as leaders can remedy this. We need to define our roles and make others aware of their responsibilities. In this way, we can hold each other accountable and spread the task load more appropriately.

4. What costs you time during the day?

Things that cost you time are processes that need to be improved. Time spent working with the EMR is so significant it will be covered separately. Other examples would be delays in rooming, late patients, missing supplies, unexpected phone calls, prior authorizations, or calls back from the pharmacy when medications are not covered. Again, if you cannot verbalize or identify these things, you cannot begin to address them.

We spend tons of time learning to interpret medical data to best help our patients, but we spend very little time analyzing how we use our time. So, *gather the data.*

REDUCE TIME-KILLERS

Here is my list of tasks that were unaccounted for in my day:

- Prior authorizations. These include paperwork or conversations with the insurance company when a service requested by the physician is not covered by the insurance, or they require more medical information before allowing the service to be covered. This was probably the biggest cost of time.

- Paperwork verifying medical condition to avoid abrupt electric or water service termination due to patient nonpayment.

- Pharmacy calls when medications are not covered by insurance.

- Other paperwork: FMLA, work excuse notes, disability forms, school physical forms.

- Duplicate forms when the patient has lost their copy.

- Medication refills for patients not in clinic.

- Calls for labs or radiology when partners or colleagues were not in office.

- Evaluations for staff and students.

Here is a list of what cost me time during the day:

- Prior authorizations.

- Unexpected walk-ins.

- Delay in rooming patients, whether due to staffing issues or patients showing after appointment time.

- Allotted appointment duration and patient expectation mismatch.
- Missing equipment during procedures.
- Clarification of clinic process to staff.
- Late staff leading to delay in huddle and start of day.
- Miscommunication of coverage.
- Unexpected illness of another provider.
- Answering questions from my APPs.
- Answering questions from my nurse.

Now that you have gathered the information, find or create a forum to discuss these problems with your team. Is everyone aware of where your (and everyone else's) time goes? And what you don't have time for?

I have found most people aren't fully aware of where their time is spent. Instead, they rush from one task to the next with interruptions all along the way. Treat time like a fixed amount of money you get every day. You can choose where you spend your time. You should budget it.

Know where you are spending your time. Without this information, you will be powerless to change your environment.

Lastly, you need a platform to discuss issues within the clinic and start incorporating these "unexpected" or "unaccounted" events into the daily clinic flow.

I have found that a team huddle prior to the start of clinic is a good forum to address any minor issues with miscommunication

REDUCE TIME-KILLERS

or small systemic issues. This is a quick 10- or 15-minute session prior to the start of seeing patients to address what patients that day need and identify potential issues.

Does your clinic carve out time weekly or monthly for larger discussions? This is an important part of improving systems.

Committee Meetings

Committee meetings are a double-edged sword. For physicians, they are an essential platform to relay input from those doing the work (physicians). But if run inefficiently, they are a huge source of time depletion.

We can do a few things to ensure our time is not wasted in yet another meeting:

- Ask for an agenda ahead of time.

- Deliberately assign action items with hard end dates.

- Limit meetings to essential personnel.

MAKE ADJUSTMENTS FOR LACK OF UNDERSTANDING FROM ADMINISTRATION

Let's shift gears from discussing administrative tasks to discussing administration. Healthcare is getting extremely complicated and there are many layers between physicians and patients. Those layers can include administrators and organizations with missions that differ from ours, especially when medical practitioners are employed instead of being primary business owners. Compounded by the evolving and increasingly influential roles of pharmaceutical and insurance companies, it seems the voices of those providing medical services and the voices of patients have been muted.

STAY IN MEDICINE

I believe physicians are in the best position to be advocates for ourselves and for patients.

We see and understand how our current system fails patients. I was speaking to a friend who just turned 26, which means he just got "booted off" his parents' health insurance. He's a healthy guy with no medical problems, working with entrepreneurs. He hunted for insurance and found he would have to pay approximately $150 a month in premiums with a whopping $8,000 deductible. My jaw just about hit the ground. He will probably not have to see a physician except for his yearly physical. He will be paying just shy of $2,000 a year, assuming he does not have to use the healthcare system. If he lands in the ER for a fracture and needs surgery, he will be expected to pay at least $10,000 before the insurance will even kick in. How does this system keep individuals healthy, medically or financially? This is just one example of how the medical system is crippling patients financially.

I understand why patients only come to me when they are on their last leg. I understand why they are so confused when they come to see me for an ankle fracture and receive inflated bills. "I have health insurance. Isn't that supposed to pay for this?" they ask.

This is where we as a system have failed. We have not kept insurance companies accountable for their subpar products, and we have not kept pharmaceutical companies or our own organizations accountable when the prices of drugs or medical services are inflated. Who else sees all of these issues and still has to look the patient in the eye? We are the only ones, as physicians and healthcare providers.

As physicians, we are the "boots on the ground." We see how fragmented this system is. It does not keep patients healthy. It incentivizes not seeking medical care. And it affects us too. It's time to challenge the system and hold it accountable. It starts with us.

HOW TO CHANGE THE SYSTEM

What can you do when there are competing missions? When what you believe and know is right for your patients conflicts with the overarching organization? How can you create change in your workplaces from any position?

Start with these basic questions and steps:

1. **Identify the decision-makers: Who ultimately makes the decisions within your organization? What does your chain of command look like? How are decisions made within your organization?**

   Often people don't know who makes the decisions in their own organization. When they make complaints, it doesn't get to the right people. Hopelessness sets in. "I brought this issue up, but nothing got done!"

   A simple solution is to create a decision-maker flow chart for everyone to see (and update it when needed).

2. **Clearly describe the problem and communicate it: Can you define the problem? Are your decision-makers even aware that there is a problem? Are the concerns of staff members going to the correct person?**

   I often see coworkers complaining to each other, but they don't elevate the issue to someone who has the power to change it. Or worse, they fail to see that they are the first step in changing the environment. Commiserating, while cathartic, is never productive. It creates a toxic environment where members feel helpless and disempowered to change their surroundings.

Articulate the problem to the right people, and don't discount that you might be the right person to start the change. Always invite your coworkers to express themselves in some way when the time is right.

3. **Be a positive role model: Don't offer complaints. Propose solutions.**

    I learned a long time ago that if you present a problem without offering a solution, others will find a solution for you. They may not have your best interests in mind or, worse, may have a poor understanding of what you do. This can lead to micromanaging or a solution that doesn't solve the problem.

    Do the research. Are there best practices? Why is your office not using them? What equipment or staffing do you need? Outline the cost along with the benefits and present them to the right decision-maker.

4. **Define the magnitude of the problem: Is this problem limited to your environment, or does it occur elsewhere?**

    Sometimes it is hard to see outside of your day-to-day when you put your head down to power through your work. Throughout our medical careers we are taught to collect and interpret data, to constantly question the medical literature, and to practice according to what evidence shows works. Yet when it comes to our business operations or clinic workflow, we do not apply the same logic. Why is that?

5. **Understand what's important to the decision-makers: Collect the right data.**

   There are two pieces of data I have found that move and shake people in administration: losing money and patient safety or satisfaction issues. Collect that data early and often.

   How much time are you spending on prior authorizations? How many adverse patient events have occurred due to overbooking, lack of appropriate staff training, or another problem you'd like to see resolved?

   We need to do more than just complain about our environments. We must continue to demonstrate how this system is hurting people.

6. **Share your findings: Share what you discover with your team, your colleagues, your administrators, and your professional organizations.**

   I have used data my team and I have collected in my previous jobs to demonstrate the need for change when I experienced hesitation from decision-makers regarding funding, time budgeting, staffing, and many other issues. I have also been able to use data I have collected on which insurance companies cost the organization time and money during negotiations. This is data we need to share with each other and is part of keeping all parties accountable.

STAY IN MEDICINE

I read an article where a physician recorded the amount of time it took to get someone on the phone to complete a prior authorization. The article went viral. As I was reading, I related personally to the frustration of the physician. How many times had I been in the same situation? How many times had I subjected my nurse to that same process in a plea for help? Weaving in and out of patient appointments, I would ask for an update and get "Nothing yet." The viral response to the article was not surprising to me. Thousands of us go through the same experience daily. Yet it's just accepted as is, and little has changed over the years. In many cases the prior authorization process has become more cumbersome. More insurance companies limit the services they are willing to pay for. Collecting that data was the start of a movement that is shedding light on the fragmented process of prior authorizations, and that data is now being used to change policy.

We have so much data about how the healthcare system hurts patients, yet when it comes to our clinics, we see the problems and simply move on. Analyze your clinic. Is this an exercise your clinic regularly does? How are systemic processes hurting your day-to-day? Which team members can help record that and how are they documenting it? Turn that data into information that matters. How much time and money are these problems costing you, your team, and your patients?

As physicians, we are in the best position to advocate for change for ourselves and for our patients. We see both sides of the coin. We see the complications when the patients cannot get the medications they need, or the delayed diagnosis when an imaging study is denied by the insurance company. We see the holes in the fabric.

When I was in medical school, I still used paper charts. I hated them. I could not read anyone's writing and I cringed when an attending would ask me to find the last CT report or last set of labs.

REDUCE TIME-KILLERS

I looked forward to the transition to electronic records. I was genuinely excited.

The creation of the electronic medical record (EMR) started with good intentions. Ultimately it was a project aimed at solving the problem of miscommunication among physicians and specialists. It was supposed to allow easier patient record transfers and translate all the hard work into a billable encounter. Yet the outcome has not been as harmonious or as efficient as I hoped.

COMMON PROBLEMS WITH THE EMR

Takes Away From Your Connection With the Patient

The EMR has the potential to interfere with the vital connection to your patients. Picture this scenario: As the patient is telling the physician what ails them, the physician is fervently trying to capture all the data.

After hearing "Uh-huh" and "Can you repeat that again?" several times, patients feel physicians are not truly listening. They are left with the impression of a cold doctor trying to move on to the next patient.

I understand why this is so. We fear not capturing all the data in the documentation for insurance reimbursements or potential litigation in the future. Not documenting in real time will mean pajama charting later or missing dinner with the family again.

Information Overload

There is so much data in the EMR that rummaging through the information costs precious time. When I want to obtain records from a specialist, if they do not share the same EMR, I still have to rely on my old fax machine for the records to be sent over for review. But now, instead of sifting through clinician notes, I'm sifting through redundant info—numerous iterations of immunization records, labs embedded in the notes, pages of mandatory questions or screening questionnaires, and patient education notes. I'm left wanting the *CliffsNotes* version of the old paper chart. A new patient visit that typically is allotted 30 minutes easily becomes overwhelming when I have to sift through pages of notes prior to even seeing the patient. This is a small example of how our current EMR adds to our already long list of things to do.

Not Necessarily More Efficient

With the rise of the EMR also came plentiful check boxes and thousands of clicks. For a time, the EMR had mandated fields that a physician had to click to get to the next screen. I cannot tell you how disruptive this was to the natural flow of a conversation with a patient. Trying to find the appropriate check box while talking to the patient quickly became too much, creating a very awkward encounter with disjointed conversation and long pauses at inopportune times.

Finding the proper fields to enter labs, referrals, and prescriptions and then link it to a diagnosis takes far longer than the old-fashioned prescription pad.

A visit with a patient may take 15-20 minutes, but at the end of the day you're committing another 15 minutes or more to document the encounter. A recent study demonstrated just this issue. According to the study, reported by the *Annals of Internal Medicine*, providers spent an average of 16 minutes in the EMR per patient encounter, and 11 percent of their time spent in the EMR was after hours (Overhage, 2020). With this occurring on an almost daily basis, it is easy to see how this time debt costs us precious moments with family and friends.

REDUCE TIME-KILLERS

Lack of Flexibility and Innovation for Practices

EMRs come in many flavors, but until you actually try a system out, you don't know what its capabilities truly are.

I have seen the implementation of three EMR platforms during my career thus far. Once you start using it, you realize the limitations some of these systems have, but then the response is, "This EMR just can't do that and we cannot change to another one because we have a contractual agreement for the next two years." So just like that, you're stuck with an inefficient system that does not meet your everyday needs for another two years. I think what adds insult to injury is witnessing the amazing technological advances in everyday life, yet not being able to do a simple task in an EMR. For example, if I buy a coffee down the street, a receipt is sent to my email in seconds, but I cannot send a patient a PDF of educational material in a secure message because the EMR does not allow it. There has to be a better way—and there is, but it costs practices a lot of money if it involves purchasing updates or a new EMR system.

The good news is using the EMR can be and needs to be a team sport. There are aspects to its use that are very beneficial. For starters, the legibility of notes and orders are far superior. Ultimately, the EMR can facilitate communication with team members and allow other ways to connect with patients.

We must continue improving EMRs and how we use them to create better efficiencies. But for now, let's concentrate on what you can control and open up the larger conversation of how you can contribute to systemic change in the future.

TIPS TO IMPROVE EMR USABILITY

Assemble Your Team

Using the EMR needs to be a team sport. One advantage of most EMRs is multiple people can document in the patient's chart at the same time. This is where the team approach will help you become a better provider and deliver better care for your patient. Everyone who works in your office is part of your team. Share the load of documentation and responsibility.

Medical assistants (MAs) can help obtain patient history and input data and your clinical note into the EMR. You may need to assist and give them some direction, but this is something they can absolutely help with. Allow team members to practice at the top of their scope and help you by lightening your burden.

Delegate Data Entry to Your Team Members

Remember those incoming records I mentioned that are faxed by another facility because you do not share the same EMR? Team members can go through the record and input the pertinent data in your current EMR in the correct areas.

- Immunization records should be transferred.

- Any previous diagnoses or surgeries should be transcribed as medical and surgical history.

- Any imaging can be scanned and placed in an appropriate folder for lab/radiology studies.

- Any cancer screenings can be identified and placed in your current EMR.

This all can and should be done before the patient sees you for their first appointment or before their follow-up appointment. In my experience in multiple clinics, there is typically no process in place to deal with information as it enters the office. This is an opportunity—this is where you must have a process, train your team, and delegate. Multiple people using the EMR works to everyone's advantage.

REDUCE TIME-KILLERS

Collaborate With Information Technology (IT)

Talk to IT right away. They are part of your team even if they may not be in the same building. If your experience was like mine, you received one or two days' training, tops, on how to use the EMR. Then you were off to the wilderness with a "call me if you need me." So that's what I did. I called a lot! And as they gave me information, I compiled the list and shared with others in my clinic. I thought everyone else just knew how to best use the EMR and I was the dummy lagging behind. Nope, that was not the case. Everyone had all sorts of workarounds to help them combat the inefficiencies they encountered at work every day.

As physicians, we are innovative. If something is not working, we will make something up to make it work. In this case, stop doing that. We were all very creative in finding ways not to use the EMR, but ultimately, it ended up costing us time or caused us to duplicate efforts. Use the experts: call IT. Show them what you do and have them shadow you. They will show you how you can do it more efficiently with the EMR. I have learned that IT really is my best friend. Many times I have been surprised by something they showed me regarding EMR.

People in IT are often one of our most underutilized team members.

We need to expand our teams and learn to truly use them. The EMR can be used to your advantage, but IT must be involved early. And not just for you as the provider, but for all your team members. If you have big plans and want to see patients in a different manner, great—get IT involved.

You can also show them what needs you have that are not currently available. This information should and must be filtered back to the software developers to continue to innovate and create EMRs that serve us better.

Use a Scribe

I'll say it again: use a scribe. Spending large amounts of time on documentation is a poor use of your time and talents. And I bet many of your team members want to serve a bigger role on your team. Here are several ways you can let them help you:

- Train your MA to be your scribe. Use a team approach to see your patients. Have your MA in the room from start to finish. The visits with the patient will be shorter, the patient will have orders completed by the time you are done talking to them, and there will be a written plan before the patient leaves your office. For this to work, you will need a 1.5 MA-to-physician ratio at a minimum.

- If you have a medical student, have them scribe several of your visits. This can become part of their learning experience and has many benefits. They get to observe how you interview patients and examine patients, and they learn how to capture key elements of the visit in a standard note. Finally, they learn the value of good communication between you and the patient and you and your team.

- If you don't have enough MAs or medical students, hire a scribe. Make sure your time is committed to tasks no one else in your office can do. Otherwise your talents are truly wasted.

- If you can't afford a scribe, use a dictation (speech to text) service. I have used Dragon in the past and even Siri.

REDUCE TIME-KILLERS

As you can see, I hate documentation and have gone to great lengths to make the EMR and documentation a team sport. With a little planning and communication, you do not have to be buried under piles of invisible paperwork.

Utilize Templates

Create macros or "dot phrases" for the most common things you do: procedures, patient education, chronic conditions, and group appointments. Create your own templates for your most common conditions. This is the sort of data you can obtain from IT. If you find yourself writing the same instructions more than once, those instructions need to be a macro or template.

I cannot emphasize enough how much of my time and effort is saved by using this method, and I can even tailor the wording to my style. I actually create "dot phrases" after I read my medical articles to ensure that the education I'm providing to my patients is the most up to date.

Have a Process for the EMR for Non-Face-to-Face Patient Encounters

These are also known to some as asynchronous visits and include portal/electronic messaging and phone messaging. These visits are not typically captured by our current models of productivity, yet they are so important. Not only do they keep patients engaged, but they also allow a venue for transfer of information without inconveniencing the patient. You need dedicated time for these.

The EMR is here to stay, so don't fight it. Use it to help you deliver the care you feel your patients need. If you have tried all the above and it's still not working, it might be time to get another system. This is where communication with IT and administration is important.

STAY IN MEDICINE

Let's take a moment to talk about workarounds to problems with EMR systems. While workarounds are good at patching up an issue at the moment, most of them do not survive the test of time. We spend a lot of time creating workarounds or relaying information to each other regarding the shortcomings of the systems we use. Yet how often do we route the information to those who have the power to change things when we cannot do it ourselves? How often do we give feedback to the companies that create and develop EMRs? Not often enough.

There is so much variability in EMRs, and yes, they do fall short in a lot of areas. When and if you have the opportunity to provide key usability feedback, provide it—even if it's unsolicited. If there are patient-related safety issues due to the EMR, raise these immediately to IT, then to the manufacturer of the software. Do not create elaborate workarounds to fix a systemic issue. This is something you can control when you do not have control of the system.

I'm hopeful that in the near future, I can get real-time information on medication coverage or when a prior authorization will be needed for a specific treatment plan through the EMR. It's an ever-evolving system that we all will need to adapt to over time.

The EMR has much potential for disease tracking among populations, zip codes, and age groups. It can help track disease in pandemics and integrate care across healthcare systems. It can also be a source to identify healthcare disparities and help with the allocation of resources to communities in need. With its use, we can deliver medicine more efficiently. Some healthcare providers have done this.

However, information is not integrated across different health systems. In fact, different health systems use different EMRs and typically there is no data integration between them. Following trends is very difficult if we remain in silos. At the clinic level, we rarely use the EMR to get to know our patient population. We often don't pause to look at trends and we don't even know the full functionality of our EMR system.

WHAT CAN WE DO WITHIN OUR OWN CLINICS?

Here are some tips to help you create more time by engaging your team to care for your patients outside of the patient visit.

Make a Contingency Plan for Unexpected Events

This needs to be done at an individual and system level. What do we do when someone calls out sick, or when we lose a member of our team for any reason? When you really think about it, being short a team member is not actually an unexpected event. It's one that many simply do not plan for. Illness and team members leaving are facts of life. Yet many organizations do not plan for this at all. Instead, everyone else "just covers," adding chaos and strain to the already difficult day-to-day. When someone unexpectedly leaves or is out for a prolonged period of time, the entire clinic suffers. There are more delays, and the time debt for those who remain in the clinic grows. There is nothing worse than being out sick for a day and coming back to a desk full of work because nothing changed in the day-to-day operations to compensate.

What is the plan when the "unexpected" happens in your clinic?

For example, if a provider is out on extended leave, a covering provider should be given dedicated time to cover these tasks.

Lack of planning for these situations eventually leads to many issues: burned-out staff, poor service and care to your patients, little time dedicated to innovation, and missed business growth opportunities for your practice.

STAY IN MEDICINE

Huddle Daily With Your Team

In our clinic, we incorporated huddles every morning with a specific agenda that I refer to as the four S's: Staffing, Schedules, Supply, and System issues. Our huddles are typically 10 to 15 minutes, and this preparation is key. This forum allows all team members to be active participants and present pertinent information as well as ensure everyone is current on the day's events.

Staffing: Who is here today? Who is covering what responsibilities for the day? This is essential for delegation of tasks.

Schedules: This is a quick review of the patients that will be coming for the day and a discussion of their needs. It allows for the appropriate schedule changes to meet the needs of the patient.

For example, if Mrs. Smith is coming in, she is 50 years old, hasn't been seen in two years, and we know she's a smoker, we can identify these things ahead of time. When she comes in, we have a list of health recommendations based on her risk factors. We might say, "Smoking increases your risk for various complications. In order to help prevent pneumonia, I would recommend a pneumonia vaccine. It also increases your risk for colon cancer—have you done your colon cancer screening already?"

If a patient's coming and we know they have a lot of needs, how can we take care of those needs without relying solely on the physicians? I regularly get my nurses and medical assistants involved. After all, they are part of the team. They can take care of issues that don't require the physician. Without allotting time for a preplanning huddle, you won't identify potential issues until the patient is in the room with the physician, and we all know how that ends . . . there is too much to address, and the appointment runs over to your next patient's appointment.

REDUCE TIME-KILLERS

Supply: There is nothing more frustrating than trying to do a procedure and finding out, while the patient is in the room, that supplies are missing. This is where your staff is key. For those who are in charge of inventory, present the information in this forum. Are there special events upcoming? Flu season? Pap nights? Upcoming deployments (for those in the military)? Is the summer over for schoolchildren and more vaccines or sports physicals will be needed? These situations impact the supply needs in your clinic and as such, should be presented in the huddle.

System issues: Are all systems operational? From computer log-ins to clinic flow, is everything functioning as it should? Discuss breakdowns in processes or flow in this forum. Were there near misses, unpleasant patient encounters, or collapses in communication? Do certain processes cost team members' time? I have found that without this forum, systemic issues are not identified or addressed in a timely manner.

While there have been many proposed agendas for a huddle, I have found the four S's to be the easiest to remember and implement. Preparation for the huddle starts before the huddle. All members of the team need to be present and ready to make their specific contribution to the four S's. After all, medicine is a team sport.

Take Time for Training

My colleagues and I would often groan over "mandatory" training. However, it wasn't until my time as medical director that I recognized how important this can be in creating a team and ensuring everyone is on the same page.

Where do we find the time for more training? First, create the time and space for this to be completed, just like you create time and space for patient appointments. Training is an essential part of your clinical operations, so treat it as such. More money and time are lost when there are unclear processes or when work is duplicated because a completed task has to be corrected. In my current practice, one to two hours per month fills this need. It is an unfair expectation for individuals to complete training on their own time at home. If it is essential to complete for clinical operations or compliance purposes, then it should be assigned during the duty day.

Second, make training pertinent to your mission, set an agenda, and make it interactive. This is not the time for death by PowerPoint. Make this time count. For topic ideas, I typically use issues that arise involving the four S's during my huddles as focal points for training as well as literature outlining best practices. Topics range from medical content, business practice updates, and professional development to team building. If time is not already carved out, make it a priority.

Dedicating time and space for training together achieves another purpose at the same time: building and nurturing a team. I regularly ask team members to present in this forum. This keeps all members engaged and assigns value to their contribution. This is an easy platform to help team members develop their soft skills. Training is crucial for keeping your clinic running smoothly, appropriately addressing issues, and ensuring everyone is practicing at the top of their game.

Delegation

How many times are you bogged down by making decisions that do not require your specific level of expertise? The only way you can practice at the top of your scope is by focusing your efforts on decisions that require your level of expertise. In turn, allow and encourage others to practice at the top of theirs. To do this, you must delegate tasks to others.

REDUCE TIME-KILLERS

Delegation starts with defining roles—starting with yours. In preparation for this, answer these two key questions:

1. What decisions/tasks require your expertise and can only be made by you?
2. What decisions/tasks don't require your expertise and can be delegated?

Begin by identifying the decisions you as the physician have to make. Those decisions are likely different than the decisions you want to make, and it's important to recognize the difference. It can be difficult to give up responsibility for some tasks, but it's necessary to preserve time for the things only you can do.

Physicians tend to be problem-solvers. It is common for many physicians to try to take everything on, including tasks that don't require your level of skill. By delegating decisions to team members who share the same mission and vision, you can focus more time on decisions only you can make. The point of this exercise is to determine which decisions can and need to be delegated.

Delegation should start with senior leadership. Name a decision that someone at the top makes. Can someone at a lower level handle that decision? If so, can someone below that person handle it? That task goes down to the next person in line and continues to be delegated as needed. We will discuss more about defining roles for each member of your team in the team culture chapter.

Make Delegation a Team Sport

Taking on tasks that your team members can handle is a massive contributor to burnout and a killer of productivity and teamwork. Get your team on board and create a unified understanding of who handles each task and decision. This creates a more efficient system for executing tasks to avoid wasting time.

This doesn't mean one person will make absolute decisions without consulting other team members. Again, it is important for all members to have a shared vision and mission. It does mean you need to delegate tasks to the team members at the lowest level and give them decision-making power within their scope.

Here's an example: If you think about this in terms of sports, the head coach on any team makes decisions on things like the final roster and the overall strategy. Lee was consulting with a youth sports team when a player brought a stray kitten into the locker room on a game day. No one knew what to do with the cat, so the head coach ended up taking half of his time organizing how to get the cat to a shelter. That task could have been delegated. Lee tried to tell the coach, "This isn't worthy of your time right now." Everyone was concerned about the cat and couldn't focus on anything else. The team lost the game, and afterward, the coach said, "You're right. I shouldn't have spent so much time on that cat." (Spoiler: the cat survived.)

It's a funny example, but this kind of situation happens all the time. Something small can eat all your time. To avoid this, everyone on the decision-making hierarchy needs to understand what their focus should be. This is especially important for patient care. If everyone doesn't play their part and take responsibility to stay focused on their tasks, the patient won't receive the best care.

Use Your Leadership Training

You likely have some leadership experience even if you've never taken a leadership course. You may have been involved in sports or the military or other leadership roles. If you haven't, seek it out. It will be one of the best investments you've ever made.

REDUCE TIME-KILLERS

TAKE 10

Make a list of the unaccounted-for tasks that eat away at your day. Then evaluate each one with this simple question: Does a physician need to do this, or could someone else on the team handle this?

Task	Requires a Physician?	Could Be Delegated?
1.		
2.		
3.		
4.		
5.		
6.		
7.		
8.		
9.		
10.		

CHAPTER 3 WRAP-UP

As a physician, you are accustomed to having many responsibilities piled on your plate. You are expected to take them on and find a way to get them all done. You can still do this without being the one to actually compete all those tasks, but it may take a deliberate effort on your part to break the habit of just doing them yourself.

Start seeing yourself not as the one who handles everything, but as the leader of a team of professionals who work together to achieve the goal of quality patient care together. It's worth the effort and time spent learning some new skills in leadership and delegation to spread the workload more evenly among your team. Evaluate each task that comes your way—especially the unplanned-for ones—and make delegating it your habit instead of just adding it to your list. You may need to train or orient people on your team to make this happen. It's worth it, if the end result is you have more time in your day to do what truly requires your skills. Plus, the result is you can go home at a reasonable hour with all your tasks completed for the day.

Join the conversation at
StayInMedicine.com

4

Refocus on Patient Relationships

> **Problem:** Healthcare systems, doctors, and patients do not share the same goals. Added expectations and requirements have eroded the physician-patient relationship.
>
> **What you control:** How you communicate with your colleagues, patients, and administrators.
>
> **Action items:** Create a daily plan for your team and start a dialogue with healthcare companies.

Loss of relationships includes the critical physician-patient relationships. Recovering those relationships requires understanding the expectations of everyone involved. Numerous expectations are put upon physicians, both by the medical system and by ourselves as physicians—not to mention the patients' expectations. Besides the pressure this creates, there is conflict when these expectations clash. Healthcare systems, doctors, and patients sometimes all have different interests and goals. Finding solutions requires communication and building relationships between all parties.

STAY IN MEDICINE

MANAGING EXPECTATIONS

Physicians and healthcare providers want to take care of their patients, and patients want to be cared for when sick. We must acknowledge that these statements mean different things for different people.

Individuals often seek our expertise in their most vulnerable moments. But in our current healthcare climate, many obstacles obscure the physician-patient relationship. There are so many expectations from both sides that it is unlikely they will all be met. And when expectations are not met, trust crumbles.

What do patients expect from the healthcare system? Most patients expect physicians to address and "fix" all their medical problems when they are first seen. At least, this is what it feels like.

Early in my career, I used to cringe when patients showed up with a full list of problems they wanted to address when they saw me for their yearly physical. After all, they waited months to see me, and to not address their problems would be perceived as negligent and callous.

But depending on the symptoms, getting to the right diagnosis often requires time and, dare I say it again, data collection. I wish I could put patients through a scanner that would give me the diagnosis. But finding out what ails a person takes time, communication, and applying logic to solve a puzzle. We must cultivate relationships and analyze tests.

Currently, it's not realistic to cover all the components of a typical wellness visit on top of an additional list of problems within 15-20 minutes.

In the U.S., healthcare is a service—not a right. While I do not agree with the way things are, this is the current situation. Often this model does not align with my mission to take care of my patients. And as with many services, you get what you pay for. In this case, patients get what their insurance company is willing to pay for.

From my personal experience as a physician and as a patient, it's clear that most individuals don't understand how insurance policies work. Physicians are expected to make decisions based on what is best for the patient. However, our decisions can result in an angry call from the patient hours later, asking why their insurance company is not willing to pay for a medical study, lab, or medication. It's frustrating for the patients and for us. Obviously, the insurance representative was not in the room when we decided on the diagnosis or treatment. The bigger problem is it's virtually impossible to know all the medications that will be covered under every type of insurance that a practice accepts.

Patients are typically unaware that most insurance plans will not reimburse physicians for addressing issues outside of the appointment. For the physician to be reimbursed for that time, the patient would have to pay additional money, according to their health insurance policy.

With the large amount of money already paid into the medical system, expectations are high. It puts both patients and physicians in a very awkward position. How can we deny needed services because we may not get paid for the work?

Your ability to be open and honest with your patients (and yourself) about their health and how the system works harkens back to the oldest and most sacred pillar of the medical profession: trust. Above all when managing expectations, create and maintain trust with your patients, staff, and team before moving on to anything else. If trust is bent or shattered, none of the rest will matter.

MISMATCHED EXPECTATIONS: THE "QUADRUPLE AIM"

Mismatched expectations or competing missions cause a variety of problems in healthcare. For example, my expectation for myself as a physician is to provide my patients with the appropriate diagnosis and treatment plan. My patient's expectation is that I keep them healthy, and this means many different things to different individuals. My organization's expectation is that I take care of the patients without losing money.

Within these three viewpoints, you can see we already have a problem. We all have different missions. In an attempt to merge our missions, some medical organizations have created the "quadruple aim" mission that many organizations have adopted to get everyone on the same page.

Here is the latest rendition of the quadruple aim as of the publishing of this book:

- **Improve patient experience.** This is typically measured by quality scores and patient satisfaction scores.

- **Improve population health.** This is measured by metrics, which in some instances may not correlate with improvement of morbidity and mortality.

- **Reduce cost.** Cost is controlled largely by insurance and pharmaceutical companies.

- **Prioritize care team well-being.** The well-being of the team is the responsibility of the individual provider. (Spoiler alert—no one tells you how to do this.)

These are the expectations set forth by large medical organizations and health systems. I agree with these goals, but the path to accomplish these goals is as nebulous as the expectations themselves. In practice, they become competing missions, and it seems physicians are the only ones held responsible for the missed expectations.

> *The reality of the medical profession today is that while we as physicians serve the well-being of the patient, medicine is also a for-profit business.*

We could write another book with the differing viewpoints on why this system is or isn't broken, but that's not the purpose of this book. **The purpose of this book is to spark conversations and make connections—relationships—that enable you to regain control over your day-to-day.**

The only way to address competing missions is to search for common ground. It's a long and often frustrating process but the needle will not move unless the conversation continues. Understand that medical organizations and health systems have a job to do also. Find out what their goals are and see if there is any potential to maximize each other's performance and find common ground.

WHAT DO WE EXPECT FROM OURSELVES?

Correct Diagnosis Every time

I expect to get the right diagnosis and treatment plan the first time I see a patient. But that is a lofty goal. Diagnosing is difficult on its own, let alone dealing with the complications we run into every day.

The following issues are typically not accounted for by patients, physicians, or organizations:

- Time constraints

- Cultural and socioeconomic differences between patient and physician
- Lack of resources and support

While these challenges are frequently discussed in medical school, there is little direction on what can be done on a practical level. No one wants to be in a position where they feel they could have done more. That's why it's so important to do everything within your power (research, questioning, follow-up, etc.) to make a correct diagnosis.

Work Completion

I was once told, "There will always be more work." Our profession proves that more than any other. While we may strive to complete all the work by the end of the day, it's impossible without a team approach. If you try to do this alone, you might as well bring a sleeping bag to the office. You must rely on your team and give yourself permission to return to the work again tomorrow when warranted.

Make a Contribution

Most physicians want to know that their work means something. We chose medicine because we care about helping people. It's easy to find yourself thinking, *Was it all worth it? The debt, time away from family and friends, the late nights studying, and worrying about a patient?*

COVID-19 proved how important physicians and other healthcare workers are to most of the world. Take solace in knowing that although there is a high cost to the lives we live, we are in a unique position to have a lasting impact on people's lives. If that doesn't motivate you, it might be time for you to reevaluate your situation.

REFOCUS ON PATIENT RELATIONSHIPS

WHAT DO PATIENTS EXPECT FROM US?

Accurate Diagnosis

The diagnosis is what patients pay for. They pay for our expertise, knowledge, and clinical acumen, and they expect our diagnoses and treatment plans to be correct and helpful. Once again, if you are doing everything within your power to make this happen, you cannot be too hard on yourself.

Positive Physician-Patient Relationship

It is no secret that the relationship between a patient and their doctor has been fragmented by pressures from the current practice of medicine. We rush from one room to another, apologetic for rushing, or apologetic for being late. Instead of "Hello," my introduction is frequently, "I'm sorry." In that rush, we forget to properly introduce ourselves, to take the time to ask how they are doing, to sit down and listen to their concerns. We easily forget we see people at their most vulnerable, and that is when they need to feel cared for most. Take a moment and collect yourself before walking into the room and provide that experience for every patient. Train your staff to limit interruptions during these visits.

Fulfilling Needs in One Visit

Medicine is expensive. I understand why patients expect to address all of their concerns at once. They are not privy to the constraints for reimbursement placed on us by insurance companies. They are there to see their doctor. Why wouldn't they ask about any healthcare concerns they have? There are too many levels of separation between the needs of the patient, care rendered, and payment.

Be open and honest with your patients about their expectations. We cannot blame them for what they don't know, but we can take time to inform them.

Coordinating Care Needs

When I put in referrals for specialty services, many of my patients frequently ask, "Is someone going to call me for an appointment with the specialist?" I don't believe patients are lazy. Most just don't know how to engage with the medical system—so you (or your team) must educate them.

WHAT DOES THE MEDICAL SYSTEM EXPECT FROM PHYSICIANS?

Always Know the Answers

As a physician, it is hard to admit when you don't know something. Over time, I have become more comfortable admitting my deficits of knowledge to colleagues and patients. Alluding to knowing more than you do is dangerous and costly to the patient. When you don't know something, do the research. With the vast advancements in medicine, it is impossible to know everything all the time.

Get the Job Done

It may sometimes feel like you must get the job done regardless of the cost to yourself. While you should do all you can to care for patients, it should not require personal sacrifice. Take the time to care for yourself. If you have a family, take the time to care for them also. It's time you cannot get back.

Be Available at All Times

Physicians are human. You need time away to recuperate and replenish. It is not possible to be always available, and you must draw a line to create time for yourself. There's a lot of talk about "mental health days" throughout our society. You deserve one once in a while too. Schedule them and keep them—don't work through them.

REFOCUS ON PATIENT RELATIONSHIPS

Meeting Expectations

How can we create an environment where everyone's expectations are at least addressed, if not met? What can we do to help moderate expectations?

Begin with these key questions to guide you in meeting expectations:

- What community do you serve? What are their needs?
- What services do you need to take better care of your patients? Is everyone involved aware of the needs of this community?
- Do you have a process when seeing patients to address expectations?
- Besides the physician, who serves your patients?
- What common problems does your community have that affect those expectations?
- What brings you meaning and/or purpose within your job?
- What do you owe yourself in order to be the best physician you can be?

PATIENT RELATIONSHIPS

Properly caring for your patients requires communicating with them. Not only do you need to know what their health issues are, you need to offer solutions that will work for them. They also need to understand your diagnosis and what their role in their own care is. Communication is improved if you have a good relationship with your patient. The less time you have with a patient, the harder it is to build a relationship with them. If your team does not support the patient's care adequately, that relationship is damaged—so team performance is a big part of maintaining good relationships.

SEVEN STEPS TO IMPROVE PATIENT CARE

1. **Remember it's all about relationships.** Because it takes your entire team to care for your patients, your relationships with your team, your administrators, and your patients all affect the outcome. Take the time to build them.

2. **Ask the patient what their expectations are for the clinic.** Ask about their expectations for their health and for you, your team, and the healthcare system you operate within, as well as the outcome of the day's visit and for the future.

3. **Communicate your expectations for your patients.** Explain to your patients your policies for providing care. Also explain the role your team plays in that care, so they understand and won't be surprised if the phone call they get doesn't come from you.

4. **Communicate your expectations for your team.** Your team should understand their roles in the patients' care and their roles in assisting you.

5. **Allow the patient to play an active role in their own care.** Offer them educational materials to help them choose the care options that will work best for them.

6. **Allow the patient to be an advocate for their own care.** Patients often don't understand the role the insurance companies play in their care options. Empower your patients to hold their insurance provider accountable when the companies fail to provide needed services.

7. **Become part of a larger movement to improve healthcare.** Ultimately, who has the responsibility to keep the patient well? We all do. Physicians can collect data on the impact of the system's policies and give that information to the parties with the power to create change.

REFOCUS ON PATIENT RELATIONSHIPS

Here is more in-depth exploration of these seven steps.

Step 1: It's all about relationships.

Take the time to get to know your staff, patients, and administrators. Because relationships enhance communication, getting to know everyone on your team, including the patient, will ease the challenge of clear communication. Your communication with your staff on behalf of the patient is as important as your communication with the patient—everyone needs to be on the same page. For details on how to do this, go to chapter 6 on team culture.

Step 2: Ask the patient what their expectations are of the health clinic.

Do you have a process to address patient expectations? During all my new patient visits, I ask three questions:
1. What is your healthcare goal for the next year?
2. How can I help get you there?
3. What result would you like from today's visit?

I want to know what their expectations are right off the bat. I get a multitude of responses, but the most common is, "I want you to listen, I want you to try your best, and I want you to give me honest advice."

However, if your patient wants something you don't offer, explain that early on. For example, if you have medical students or residents in the clinic and your patients do not agree with the care team, tell them early on so the patient can make the decision on whether or not your clinic is a good fit for their needs.

Step 3: Outline expectations for patients.

I frequently tell my patients, "I serve as a guide for your healthcare, but ultimately your health is your responsibility. You are in control of your own ship. I will present what I know from the data, but the decision is yours and I will respect that decision."

What happens when a patient does not follow your treatment plan? I firmly believe in shared decision-making and in motivational interviewing. But some patients will disagree with you or need more time. This is hard in a system that penalizes providers when diabetics' A1C results are not within goal—or when outcomes of surgeries or procedures are completed without accounting for the patients' risk factors leading to the procedures. While I may get penalized for not meeting metrics, I don't fire patients from my practice if they do not follow the recommendations I give them. However, I do ask them if they feel I am the right doctor for them.

What expectations do you have for your patients? Set these expectations with your patients early. If there are late policies or policies surrounding controlled substances, let those processes be known early.

I use a team approach when caring for patients, so I tell my patient up front that they will receive phone calls from my staff since they are part of the care team. My staff helps to deliver care or responses regarding labs or other medical information in a timely manner. I use care coordinators and scribes as well, and I find most patients are okay with these processes if they're explained up front. I even engage my team to help patients meet their goals with check-ins and timelines. These efforts are typically well received and lead to better health outcomes for patients.

Step 4: Outline expectations for your healthcare team.

Make expectations clear to your team with specific job descriptions and a forum for debriefs. No one can meet expectations if they don't know what the expectations are. Resentment builds over time when this step is skipped.

You need the proper channels for effective communication. If you can't identify the proper channels in your current system, they need to be created. You need a forum to discuss when expectations are not being met. This can be part of daily huddles and weekly or monthly staff meetings.

Above all, make sure that anyone you work with has a clearly defined role. The alternative is having people show up to work each day with no direction, drive, or discipline.

Step 5: Allow the patient to fulfill an active role in their medical care.

I frequently give patients medical literature to read. In a span of 15-20 minutes, we often have little time or space for patient questions or a way for the patient to weigh which medical treatment option is best for them. So they get homework, but in return they get to be part of the decision process to choose their medical therapy. They get to read about the options and pick their treatment. I find they are happier doing this.

I may not see things that are important to my patients. For example, some people are bothered by a medication that makes them urinate more or a medication that gives them dry mouth. I have patients who would rather have surgery and others who would do everything humanly possible to avoid procedures.

We can and should give them that choice.

Step 6: Allow the patient to be an advocate for their own care.

Teach patients to be advocates for themselves.

What financial entity provides services to the patient? As a physician, you have the information regarding the patient's medical needs and how and why these needs are not being met. In most other industries, people understand the product they are buying and what the absolute cost is. But with health insurance, most patients do not understand the product they have bought until they try to use it. They don't understand until they attempt to fill a prescription or suddenly fall ill and cannot get the services they need due to lack of coverage.

Who holds insurance companies and health systems accountable when the population they serve does not get the services they need? Insurance is supposed to provide a service. As a system, we need to hold them accountable. And it has to start with the consumer of these services (the patient), followed by the recipient (those who provide the services).

Involve the patient in the process. I frequently have patients call their insurance companies when medications are not covered or three-way the patient during peer-to-peer conversations when imaging is not authorized. In the age of social media, no one wants bad press, and everyone has a voice that can be heard by thousands. Empower your patient to hold their insurance company accountable when they fail to provide services that are needed. If insurance is offered as part of an employer compensation package, have them file a complaint with HR. This feedback is crucial to changing the current system. How can we keep patients healthy or appropriately care for them when vital laboratory, radiologic studies, or medications are denied or not covered?

As it stands, as a primary care physician, if a patient has severe abdominal pain and I want to order a STAT CT, it is easier for me to send the patient to the ER to get certain studies done than ordering one out of my office. The current system not only dissuades physicians from ordering studies that are essential, it also makes the patient jump through hoops to get those tests. This often costs them more money (especially if they have to go to an ER to get the study approved) or encourages them to delay a diagnosis or care.

REFOCUS ON PATIENT RELATIONSHIPS

Another way we can show patients how to advocate for themselves is to have them ask for transparency. This means asking for price transparency regarding medical services including appointments, procedures, medications, and lab tests. Patients typically don't know how much a procedure or service will cost prior to getting an appointment or filling a prescription. Many just ask if the insurance will cover it. But in current times when medical bills are a joint expenditure, it is important to ask how much these services will cost before they are rendered, when possible. If this is not possible due to an emergency, then it is important for patients to ask for an itemized bill.

Legislation outlined in the Public Health Services Act, under the Affordable Care Act, now requires hospitals to disclose usual pricing for healthcare services. More legislation is underway, prompted by a presidential executive order signed in June 2019, with a particular focus on transparency with health insurance companies and their related services (45 *CFR* Parts 147 and 158, 2019). The proposal will mark requirements for group health plans and health insurance issuers to disclose cost-sharing information upon request. While not perfect, this is a start . . . but ultimately the patient will need to be proactive, engaged, and involved.

I would argue that many physicians don't truly know the cost of healthcare. We have been left out of that conversation for many years. As individuals, we would be appalled if we were expected to pay for a house renovation without a quote given ahead of time. Imagine if you were expected to pay for a meal while being completely blind to the cost. In our current system, this is what patients are expected to do.

For employed physicians, how much does your organization charge for the services you perform? If you don't know, it's time to ask. This has been a key deficit in holding our own organizations accountable.

If you don't take the steps to enable your patients, their blame will often fall back on you as the physician.

Learn to Be an Advocate for Yourself

If some issue or circumstance in your clinic prevents you from doing your job, find a way to start discussions on process improvements. It's understandable that sometimes it's easier to just take care of things yourself. When you do that all day, it adds up and can become a source of resentment and burnout.

Literature suggests if 20 percent of your time is spent on work you find meaningful, it is enough to "fill your bucket" (Herrera, 2019). If this is the case, with the understanding of the immense problem with physician burnout, why is this not integrated into the job/career landscape with medical organizations across the board? For now it's up to us, so find work that is meaningful to you and fight for it.

Step 7: Become part of a larger movement to improve healthcare.

Ultimately, who has the responsibility to keep the patient well? We all do.

All parties involved must accept their responsibility to create systemic change. When insurance companies are not willing to pay for services or when they require long approval processes, it creates problems for patients and physicians. When organizations have high profit margins on services rendered, the patients pay a high price. As a society, we foot the bill in the prevalence of illness.

I don't have an answer to these problems, but the conversations around them need to continue and, if anything, ramp up. As physicians, we need to do what we do best: collect data and give that

REFOCUS ON PATIENT RELATIONSHIPS

information to parties that have the power to create change. This starts in our respective clinics and hospitals.

We can start with ourselves. We are the experts in the field, and we can help others recognize these systemic issues and propose solutions. Have constructive conversations and debates with your colleagues with the goal of making our system better.

TAKE 10

In Step 2 of the steps to improve patient relationships, I shared the three questions I ask my patients to understand their expectations. Take 10 minutes to come up with the questions you would like your patients to answer about their expectations for you, your team, and their health.

1.

2.

3.

REFOCUS ON PATIENT RELATIONSHIPS

CHAPTER 4 WRAP-UP

You, your patients, your employer, the insurance companies, and your team members all have expectations for the outcome of the work you do. These expectations can be in conflict, making finding common ground challenging. Insurance companies' requirements can restrict your ability to provide quality care for your patients. We all have a role to play in making this system better, starting with building relationships with everyone involved to improve communication.

The limited time you have with your patients makes it necessary to have a plan for how you will learn their expectations and build that relationship with them.

Join the conversation at
StayInMedicine.com

5

Find Connection to Reframe Physician Isolation

"Don't set yourself on fire trying to keep others warm."
—Penny Reid

> **Problem:** Physicians feel isolated due to the constraints of their jobs and the lack of supportive community.
>
> **What you control:** The effort you make to connect with colleagues and the time you set aside for personal relationships.
>
> **Action item:** Recognize that asking for support from your team is not an admission of weakness. It is a request for assistance in achieving the common goal of patient care. Define the roles of your team members and ensure everyone is on board with the collective mission to build a better community of support. Schedule time for connection with colleagues.

A colleague of mine in residency referred to medicine as a mistress, always demanding of your time and killing relationships with family, friends, and partners. At the time, I thought that was a ridiculous and awkward analogy. But he was right. Cultivating relationships takes time and effort. When you spend all your time in the clinic, it's hard to keep relationships outside of medicine. It's also hard to keep relationships strong within the medical community when you rarely can spend time to maintain them.

In my mind, the largest contributors to physicians' feelings of isolation are time constraints, lack of help, and loss of relationships. Many medical professionals and organizations have weighed in on this topic (Masters, 2019; Pearl, 2019; Rubin, 2016).

In my professional and personal search, I have come to this conclusion: all of the causes of physician isolation are symptoms of systemic problems in medicine. This does not mean we are helpless. Change must begin somewhere, and it can start with physicians and our teams.

ENGAGE YOUR TEAM TO PREVENT TASK OVERLOAD

For many physicians, the care of patients feels like a constant battle against time—staying on time, finding time, and making time. For me, the days were relentless. And to top it off, the words of my previous mentors echoed in my head: "You need to make time to call that patient back," or "Find time to look that issue up." But we're only allotted 24 hours a day, and hopefully at least six are committed to sleep.

I felt alone in my battle against time, even though my colleagues were fighting the same battle. I never gave myself the opportunity to analyze what was going on or how to fix it. Eventually, I had an epiphany: Everyone I worked with was also allotted only 24 hours in a day. Why was I still at work after 6 p.m., and where did everyone else go? We were supposed to be a team, but my time investment was so much higher than the rest of my team. I felt constantly left behind.

FIND CONNECTION TO REFRAME PHYSICIAN ISOLATION

Don't allow your team to let you handle all the work.

Physicians spend much more of their time working than anyone else on the team. As a physician, you don't even have enough time to take care of all the important things that need to get done. Don't allow tasks you don't have time for to fall onto your plate—delegate them to someone who can handle them.

YOU ARE NOT AN ISLAND—ASK FOR HELP

The lack of help physicians experience is both perception and reality. But I want to focus on two general ways you may experience lack of help: the feeling you should not or cannot ask for help, and the lack of staffing to help with the work.

The first is a perception that others cannot help us, or adversely, our reluctance as physicians to seek help. This is something embedded in our culture and for me, specifically, it stemmed from frequently being told, "This is something you should know so you don't kill a patient."

The work culture constantly reminds us that the stakes are high. We often berate fellow physicians or medical students when they're not familiar with a subject—it's a learned behavior. Early in my career, this kind of culture kept me from asking for help. Instead, I felt I needed to read more or commit myself more. I felt alone—an imposter. Years later, I discovered many other physicians felt the same. That realization was as much a relief as it was an annoyance. It goes to show that if we would just have the conversations, we would be in a better place. Instead we are slowly creating a toxic culture of resentment that will result in being eaten alive. We have to be better than that.

We also experience a physical lack of help for all the tasks we are expected to complete. Our current business models focus on face-to-face time with patients and neglect the work behind the scenes. And worse yet, in spite of being part of a team, most of the work outside of face-to-face appointments is funneled to the physician.

As a student, how was I supposed to know the lack of help I'd have when I became a physician? I kept my head down, trying to complete the work I'd been taught was solely mine.

For every encounter with a patient, a physician spends about 30 minutes documenting the encounter. As stated earlier, it's notoriously called "pajama time," when we spend at least one or two hours a night just documenting.

There must be a team approach to address all the additional tasks physicians face.

Chapters 3 and 6 provide tools and suggestions for some ways to do this. If you find a successful way of doing this in your clinic, spread the word (my email address and Facebook page are at the end of this book) in any way you feel will benefit others.

LOSS OF RELATIONSHIPS

The loss of relationships physicians experience is broad. It encompasses the lack of relationships with patients, the lack of relationships with colleagues, the loss of personal relationships, and the loss of your relationship with yourself.

Patients

Medicine is all about relationships. At least, it is supposed to be. The relationship with a patient is sacred. I have helped care for patients in all socioeconomic walks of life, in times of joy and tragedy and heart-wrenching suffering. My insurmountable workload fractures these relationships. While I'm talking to a patient, my task box fills up with requests for call-backs, laboratory study reviews, medication refill requests, insurance denial claims that now need appeals or authorization forms, and the list keeps going.

Appointment time constraints do not allow me to fully address the patient's needs or questions while also fulfilling health insurance requirements. There is so little flexibility in our schedules that any small change or additional request will make you late. When your patient comes in for her well woman exam and you discover she has severe depression, you are at a precipice. Do you open Pandora's box because it is best for the patient, knowing you probably will not make it to dinner with your family?

Over time, it becomes easy to resent your patients. This is why budgeting time and focusing only on what you can control are so vital.

Colleagues

During medical school, I was encouraged to find mentors and discuss the challenges of medicine with fellow colleagues. During residency, there was a forum for the same. But when I became an attending doctor, that network disappeared. If you do get the chance to chat with your colleagues, it's typically between appointments or when rushing to lunch, and it can seem like a commiserating session. And it stops there.

As it stands, there is no time carved out to analyze what's going on, find the root of a problem, or make a strategic plan to fix things. By the time you are done seeing patients, there is a long list of tasks waiting for you, and most of your staff is gone for the day. You must decide whether to go home and finish the work there or just stay at work a little longer and plough through. When you feel burned out, how do you find the time to share those feelings with anyone else?

This is why it's so important that clinics and healthcare systems make it a point to do team-building sessions on a regular basis. There are multiple professional consultants who specialize in team building. Making time in the schedule for team-building training and events is a good investment for all parties involved.

Spouse or Partner

Medicine is a lifestyle marked with sacrifice, not just for physicians, but for all the members of their families. This was the biggest surprise for me. I didn't account for how much time it would take away from my family. The senior resident who compared his experience with medicine to a perpetually unsatisfied mistress made my jaw drop. Tears in his eyes, he described the unhealthy relationship he had with medicine, how it tore his family apart and left him lost. I judged him that day. I had no idea what he was referring to and felt the comparison was over the top. I get it now.

It's difficult for spouses when you're missing a large portion of not just each other's lives, but also your children's. This is a reality for many physicians. Most rationalize this by saying, "This is why we are compensated so highly." If your definition of success is based on income alone, true happiness will be an unfortunate sacrifice.

This isolating and unbalanced lifestyle is also a leading cause of the trending exodus of physicians from medicine.

As a female physician, there was another element that added to my feeling of isolation. For Lee and me, my career has also required an adjustment to the traditional gender and family roles.

> *For female physicians, there's the unspoken pressure of an ultimatum: your career or your family life.*

FIND CONNECTION TO REFRAME PHYSICIAN ISOLATION

I've heard countless stories from my colleagues of being passed up for promotion as they entered maternity leave or feeling forced to go part time due to inflexibility or lack of control over schedules.

When Lee and I were dating, the first thing I told him was, "I'm going into medicine." And then I hit him with the second slap, which was, "I'm joining the military." This meant he was going to be in for a life where I was constantly drawn away from family with inflexible work hours, deployments, and forced moves at least every three to four years.

I can't even imagine what was going through his head when we were so early in our relationship. But I had made a choice. I had to be a doctor.

More than a decade later, I see the same concerns with the students and residents who rotate through my clinic. Where is the balance between this life and the one at home?

Lee had his own goals and dreams he wanted to pursue. He understood and admired my passion and drive to reach my goal and I admired his. We decided to take the plunge together and never looked back.

We are very fortunate. I know there are homes where this is not possible. If we value a physician's thoughts and opinions, as a system, we can be more flexible to ensure that we don't handicap our colleagues who have families or obligations outside of work.

I was able to find a group of women battling the same issues—the Physician Moms Group (PMG) on Facebook. Check them out. I was able to learn from these very successful women who are "doing it." Through them, I realized that my mom guilt was not mine alone, and I learned how to recruit help and how to reexamine relationships.

Investing in relationships and support systems at home has been crucial. Lee has been essential for combating my physician isolation. To make our relationship work and grow, I had to recognize that Lee's life as a husband supporting his doctor wife was not easy for him either. We have always been clear with each other about our goals, our fears, our concerns, and everything in between. We established trust as our foundation, and we are mutual benefits to each other. Stepping forward together meant we had to communicate, challenge perceived notions of gender roles, and focus on our commitment to our children and each other.

As Lee often says, "It's about the we, not the me."

Sense of Self

After spending so much time studying and working, there is very little time for self-care. Your evenings may be devoured by "pajama time," documenting the encounters of the day. It can be difficult to even find time to use the restroom during a busy day at the clinic. The lack of regard for your own well-being can begin to undermine your sense of self. When you're constantly putting your own needs aside to help others, you neglect your own physical, mental, and emotional heath. It's no wonder physicians feel burned out.

> *How can you provide care for others if you cannot take care of yourself? You can't give someone something you don't have.*

As a system, we are so focused on decreased patient encounters leading to decreased revenue that we don't account for physicians burning out and leaving medicine. Per a study conducted by Stanford, the Mayo Clinic, and the American Medical Academy (Shanafelt et al., 2019), the cost of physician turnover and decreased work hours due to burnout costs $3-6 billion a year. Currently 300-400 physicians a year take their lives, which is 40 percent higher

FIND CONNECTION TO REFRAME PHYSICIAN ISOLATION

for male physicians and 130 percent higher for female physicians compared to the general population.

300-400 lives.

$3-6 billion a year.

Do I have your attention?

This is a systemic issue.

So how do we find time and help? How do we reconnect?

A focus on relationships is key. Investing in your "non-medical" relationships, family, and self are extremely important. However, every family situation is unique and it would be presumptuous for us to try and tackle the complexities of relationships in this book. For that reason, the remainder of this chapter will focus on how to create a supportive work environment and medical culture. Some of these concepts have been discussed in earlier chapters, but we have summarized them here for review.

STEPS TO OVERCOME ISOLATION
Step 1: Build a Community at Work

A team approach is essential to caring for patients and caring for each other as colleagues.

Define your collective missions. A community must have common ground, so let's find it. You can start with simple questions: What is our mission? Is everyone working toward that mission? For administrators, do your patients know what your mission is?

My mission is to take care of my patients and to operate without a loss while doing so.

For the organization to be successful, the mission must be the same for everyone—from hospital administrators all the way down to medical technicians. It is easy for providers to be stuck between competing missions: delivering healthcare and making money.

Define roles. Does everyone know what they are supposed to do? Does everyone know what everyone else does?

Look at everyone's roles and responsibilities. What are their roles? Are they living up to them? Include the patients—ultimately their health is their responsibility. They have a crucial role.

List the tasks and split them up. What is the work that needs to get done to complete the mission, and who is currently doing it? Are they the right people for the job?

Delegate the work to team members according to their roles and responsibilities. Caring for patients is a shared responsibility. It starts with administration and runs all the way down to housekeeping. It's time to adopt this thinking and embrace it across the board.

For physicians, what work are you currently doing, and can some of this work be done by someone else on the team?

Work like a community. Create a clear workflow for all of the tasks. These items should be accounted for during the workday. If a task was not accounted for, it can be the start of the organization's next process improvement project.

Step 2: Reallocate Time

Treat time like money. Time needs to be budgeted and properly allocated. And once the time is spent, it's gone. Designate time for communication among team members. Just like sports teams, practice and discuss strategy before playing the games.

Allocate time for communication. Effective communication requires intention and an agenda.

   a. **Start with a daily huddle.**

      Start with a 15-minute block of time every day that's dedicated to strategizing. Huddles should be nonnegotiable.

FIND CONNECTION TO REFRAME PHYSICIAN ISOLATION

Everyone needs to participate. Make decisions for the day during the huddle. There is nothing worse than being interrupted while talking to a patient, especially for situations that could be anticipated.

b. **Protect time for training and teaching staff.**

How often do you fix the same problem over the course of a month, or a year? These inefficiencies add up. Proper training can prevent repetitive work. Make this part of your clinic's health maintenance, not a reactive, urgent session when something goes awry.

c. **Protect time for analysis of workflow and ideas for improvement projects.**

When you implement an improvement project, retrieve data to see if the implemented changes worked. Currently in the medical industry, it seems we use scientific reasoning for all we do except daily workflow. Use scientific methods to improve your processes and to see if your improvements are helping or not.

Recruit help. When allocating time to communicate is not enough, find help to lighten the burden. Look in the literature. What has been demonstrated to save time? Here are a few ideas:

a. **Employ scribes.**

This is one way to transfer some of your workload and more effectively engage your patients.

b. **Use macros for electronic health records.**

Approach your use of the EMR with an analytical mindset and identify commonly repeated processes. Get IT help or whatever you need to streamline these processes.

c. **Train your staff and enable them to perform at the top of their skills.**

Empower your people with decision-making tools and information. They may still need to consult you on some things, but if they handle 90 percent of the effort for a task you used to do yourself, it's a win.

d. **Allow flexibility in scheduling patients.**

It's time to rethink our business model in medicine. Business meetings occur through videoconferencing, so why do we always require patients to be seen in person?

As a result of the pandemic, the use of telemedicine has exploded. Personally I have found more pros than cons. The number of patients that "no-show" to a telemedicine appointment is minimal. And I can see patients in their environment, in the comfort of their homes, and address the majority of their issues. Yet this is a mode of delivering care that medicine was slow to adopt. We need to be part of the effort to decrease barriers. We need to embrace more innovative ways to engage with patients and their communities.

Step 3: Reinvest in Relationships

Relationships are what will save healthcare. Currently there are many barriers to building good relationships. How can we create a platform to reconnect?

Get to know your colleagues. Create networking events between departments and make a point to reach out to your colleagues. These can be scheduled events or something as small as checking in with a colleague from time to time. You would be surprised how crucial these interactions are for laying the foundation of a relationship you may have to lean on during times of crisis.

FIND CONNECTION TO REFRAME PHYSICIAN ISOLATION

Get to know your patients. Over the last several years, I have made a point to get to know the people I give advice to. Chit-chat is important and doesn't take much effort. Share decision-making with the patient. I often ask my patients, "What is your health goal for this year?" After all, it's their health on the line. In getting to know your patients, you can devise plans that fit with their lives and that they can adhere to.

Within organizations, assign mentors and mentees. Take the military approach. I was very fortunate to be part of an organization where mentorship was an expected part of everyone's job—so much so that this was assigned. While my time in the U.S. Air Force was one of the hardest in my career, I didn't feel as alone as I do outside the military. From day one, you were assigned a sponsor who introduced you to the clinic or the Air Force base. They gave you the lay of the land. Once you were integrated into the clinic, you were introduced as a member of a team . . . and it felt like a true community. We were accustomed to mentoring one another and we actively looked for opportunities for promotion or career progression not just for ourselves, but also for others. Mentoring was just part of the fabric and time was allocated for such.

Promotion was an expectation for everyone, and mentorship was part of what was expected to get everyone promoted. As officers, we were not only mentors for each other, but also for our young airmen. We all frequently worked together on process improvement projects and provided advice on how to balance a full-time job and school, which a lot our young airmen did.

If mentorship is not already an expectation in your organization, you can create it. This is something we can definitely learn from the military.

Create a structure to share ideas and projects. It is understandable that many feel creativity is stifled in medicine right now . . . in part because it is. Especially for those of us who are very much clinical (meaning most of our days are spent exclusively seeing patients). When is there time to problem-solve on a system level or even work on projects that you want to do? Do you even know what active projects are ongoing in your organization?

How does your organization encourage creative thinking or idea sharing? Or do they discourage it?

For many of us, discussing new ideas or the "latest and greatest" from reading a journal article is rare. Often it only happens if we have time to go to a live conference or are presenters of poster presentations.

I was recently in a situation where I didn't find out a colleague was working on a project until the day she was expected to make the formal presentation for it. I work with her all the time—how did that happen? I said, "That was a cool project. I would have totally helped you if I had known you were working on it." It was a missed opportunity on both ends.

The good news is we can create these platforms within our organizations. We can incorporate these discussions into the fabric of the day-to-day.

Is there a platform within your organization for discussing who is working on current projects, or what projects are open and looking for volunteers? Is this announced in department meetings or faculty meetings? This kind of practice could be put in place in your organization to foster idea sharing and creativity. It doesn't have to require a complete upheaval of the current flow or, worse yet, another independent meeting.

I have also found that social media platforms are incredible for idea sharing in medicine. I remember a point in my career where social media was considered unorthodox and discouraged. But for many of us, it is a window into how others practice medicine. I can

FIND CONNECTION TO REFRAME PHYSICIAN ISOLATION

see what my colleagues are doing in academics, private practice, research, etc. Groups such as the Physician Moms Group (PMG) on Facebook and its subgroups have been a great resource to finding best practices or even tangible ideas for troubleshooting issues within my clinic. It has given me access to individuals I would have never encountered through the traditional networking events or venues. Fostering communities and platforms like this can help us and expand our roles to collaborate with others.

Create a shared conscience. Be kind and share successes and failures with each other to change the current medical culture.

I cannot emphasize this enough: Help and let others help you. As a physician leader, it is okay to show your vulnerability. I have started meetings with, "Well, that didn't quite work how I wanted. Let's regroup." I have also pointed out the successes of others as part of the huddle. It is through sharing our successes and failures that others learn. It also creates an opportunity for others to acknowledge and share as well.

Reach outside of your local network using social media. With the advent of social media, forging new relationships and networks with similar interests has become easier. The world truly has become smaller. And your access to information and expertise is easier than ever.

I saw the potential social media offers after my family was on the receiving end of the destruction Hurricane Maria brought to Puerto Rico. My family lives in a rural area with very limited resources and they were left without running water and electricity, as well as other necessities. Within weeks of the hurricane, I reached out to experts through social media to figure out how I could help. In a short time, I was able to collect three pallets' worth of relief supplies, raise funds, ship, and distribute those supplies—all thanks to the collective "how-to guide" provided by individuals I had never met.

Social media can be a great tool for mentorship, information gathering, or dissemination of much-needed education. As a medical community, it is time we embrace this.

Support each other as physicians. Social media has been a life changer for me and for many female physicians. Personally, balancing being a mother, wife, healer, and educator is a constant juggling act. Through social media, I have been able to find a community that understands the struggles of being a physician. It has been a place where I find inspiration and comfort as I read stories of others struggling with the same issues.

For me, formal networking events are sometimes difficult and time consuming. As a physician that is constantly mindful of where I spend my time, social media has allowed me to network without sacrificing time with my family.

Employer-sponsored networking or collaboration events may be beneficial, especially if they provide time during your workday to attend (West et al., 2014).

FIND CONNECTION TO REFRAME PHYSICIAN ISOLATION

TAKE 10

Take an honest look at your daily and weekly social interactions to find places for intentional improvement.

1. How would you rank your interaction with your loved ones at home? What would an ideal situation look like?

2. How often do you get a chance to talk "shop" with other physicians and medical professionals? If you don't have a daily huddle with your own team, this is a place to start. What would be an ideal arrangement for you, beyond the daily huddle?

CHAPTER 5 WRAP-UP

Physicians need to interact with other physicians to share experiences and ways to improve. Medicine is about relationships, both in practicing it for the benefit of patients and as a fulfilling profession. Evaluate your degree of isolation and take deliberate steps to improve your connections.

No physician can be an island and the current demands of medical practice make it nearly impossible to practice without the support of your team. Engage your team to improve patient care and for your own benefit. Engage in relationship-building conversations with your patients as well. Make a habit of asking about others' lives during professional, patient, and team member interactions. As a system, we can weave this into the fabric of our clinics.

Join the conversation at
StayInMedicine.com

6

Create a Team Culture

Problem: Most medical clinics lack a positive team culture to support physicians, team members, and patients.

What you control: How you interact with team members, the expectations you set for them, and the environment you create around you.

Action items: Hold team members accountable for their duties, improve communication, and invest in team-building activities to foster a better team environment. Develop your leadership skills to accomplish these goals.

It's clear that your burden of work as the physician could be eased by creating a better-functioning team approach to the work. There are too many tasks that currently fall to the physician, many of which can be handled by someone without a medical degree. Let's examine once again how the prevalent culture in medicine does not foster a team environment.

- The responsibility of all medical care falls on the shoulders of the physician.

- Time allocation is unequal between tasks and between team members.

- Roles and responsibility are unclear for many team members.

I have been in situations where the clinic environment was hostile—where there were no processes for booking patients, seeing patients, or addressing simple questions. After a long day of clinic, you may get back to your desk and find there are too many team members looking for directives from you. After working in four clinics in very different geographic locations and settings, my conclusion is that dysfunctional clinics are more the norm than the exception.

Moreover, as a physician, you cannot always be available to answer questions without compromising your personal life and ultimately impacting the way you care for your patients. If a patient walks in and asks to speak to you, it is not fair to the patient you are currently seeing if your staff interrupts the visit to get the question answered. Develop processes for these circumstances and communicate them to your team.

I have outlined in this book how there are just too many tasks for one person to complete. That situation is often made worse where there is no team structure and no sense of shared responsibility from other members in the clinic or organization.

Creating this team environment and shared responsibility for patient care is a goal you can strive for within your current clinic structure, and it can ease your workload and stress. It may also create a more positive working environment for you and everyone on your team.

Medical care should be (and is better when) delivered by teams.

CREATE A TEAM CULTURE

Building and maintaining a successful and efficient team can be challenging, but it is not impossible. This chapter will lay the groundwork for you to achieve this for yourself.

Once, I walked into a new job where the staff all had different motives. Some were committed to their work, some were only there to collect a paycheck, and others were just lost. There was no sense of community, shared responsibility, or camaraderie. "That's not my job," was recited repeatedly, words that for me are like nails on a chalkboard. As 4:30 p.m. hit, half the staff left while others were drowning in tasks. The resentment and hostility between team members was immense. I have seen similar scenarios play out in various environments in medicine.

Coming from the military where camaraderie and teamwork were instilled in everything we did, it was hard to integrate into a practice that did not have these things in place. I was trying to see patients while creating workarounds for all the deficits in the clinic. When a leadership opportunity opened, I ran to it. I knew if things did not change, I would not survive that job.

HOW TO CREATE A CLINIC TEAM

In the first few weeks as the new director of the clinic, I had everyone complete a workflow survey I obtained from the AAFP (American Academy of Family Physicians), assessing the various aspects of our organization:

- Standard operating procedures
- Decision-making structure
- Organizational structure
- Authority and chain of command
- Teamwork

- Communication

- Mission

- Camaraderie

If you want to use this survey in your own clinic, you can find it at the AAFP's website (https://www.aafp.org/fpm/2008/0500/p23.pdf).

Unsurprisingly, we fell short in all the categories. When I first came to this clinic, I had all the optimism in the world, only to become deflated, frustrated, and overwhelmed. I realized two things immediately:

1. The military was a role model for how to create high-functioning teams.

2. I didn't know how to create a high-functioning team in my current environment.

The reality is, there's a lack of understanding of the importance of teamwork within the medical profession. Teamwork in medicine is not a new concept. There is plenty of literature outlining a team approach leading to improved patient outcomes in high risk settings, like trauma. Yet this is not applied to many of the realms in medicine.

The first step is reigniting the belief that working together toward a common goal is simple and essential. It will make people feel better about themselves, about each other, about the workplace, and about their practice. It gives you a reason to wake up the next day and move forward.

Any group of people who can commit together to a common goal has a much higher chance of succeeding than groups who don't. Almost everyone, whether they're introverts or extroverts, wants to be part of something bigger than themselves.

CREATE A TEAM CULTURE

To accomplish this, there must be team buy-in and accountability. These are essential in order to create a team culture. You're not just accountable for your own actions, but for those of the team as a whole. At face value, this seems like a simple concept, however it is a skill set very few possess—how to create a team structure when one does not exist, and how to sustain that team. But it is the key to improving your day-to-day experience because teams accomplish more together.

ESTABLISH TRUST

How to you build a team? You have to start with the foundation.

The foundation of a team is trust.

To build trust, you must have some kind of relationship with each person on your team. Relationships enhance communication and help your team understand what's important to you and help you understand what's important to them.

Trust is more than simply relying on someone else. In your clinic, it may mean not going behind each other's back and not commiserating. You don't have to like everybody you work with in order to trust them. There's a difference between liking and respecting/trusting someone. You might not hang out and get a drink after work. If you trust and respect someone, you know that person is doing everything they can to achieve the same thing you are. Of course, if drinks are a welcome option, go for it.

To work together well, everyone must have an understanding of trust and what it means to everybody in that clinic. Without trust, no environment where people are asked to work together will succeed. Together, define what the word means to your team and how you're going to enact it.

Lee always says this about teamwork to the sports and business teams he works with: "When a group of individuals can bond together to accomplish a common goal, it's a miracle. Create miracles daily!"

The medical clinic environment consists of teams within teams. The physicians are a team and the nurses are a team, but you're all part of a bigger team. How all of that works together is an art and a science.

Team development is essential to move forward, but how many of us know how to actually do this? People are quick to say they don't have the time. If you do not commit time to investing in team building, you are truly wasting valuable time and resources in the long run. In the medical world, we must dedicate time or find someone externally to help create a team structure. Only a team structure can develop your common vision and goals and define your path forward as a group.

Create a Team Bond

Creating a team bond is not difficult. Maintaining it is the hard part. There are experts who can help you with this if you don't feel you have the knowledge or time to take this on—*it's that important.* Even if you cannot spend a lot of time on it, any time you spend on team development will help. And you must do it consistently and with purpose.

While every team is different, there are some cornerstones you can start building now to begin establishing a bond. The strategies in this book all correspond to creating a great clinic, and here's how they correspond to creating a great team.

1. Define your common purpose.

Vision, mission, objectives, and tactics. If you are going to work together effectively, everyone needs to be on the same page. Does

CREATE A TEAM CULTURE

everyone know the organization's vision and mission? If not, literally write it on the wall. It is that important. Without this crucial step, you cannot move forward.

Vision (long-term plan): The core of what you are trying to accomplish during your tenure as a leader. For example, Disney's vision is "to make people happy." What is the overall goal?

Mission (1-2-year plan): Clear and succinct answers to the following questions for your team's current mission: Who? What? When? Where? Why? How?

Objectives (month to month): Major actions that will be accomplished within a 1-2-year time frame. Who is responsible for it, when it will be accomplished, and the metric/metrics that define success.

Tactics (day to day): The daily, weekly, and/or monthly tasks that align to the objectives that must be accomplished.

We will explore these elements in more depth.

2. Define roles and responsibility.

What is everyone's role in fulfilling the common purpose? This is where the job description is crucial. As an initial exercise, I had all of the staff, including myself, write their own job description as they understood it. Then I compared it with the real job description, if it existed. Most of my team members were not aware of one or more things that fell in their scope of responsibility.

Without this step, no one knew what to expect from each other. I also discovered a lot of my members did not know what their colleagues did or what programs were their responsibility. Team members did not know who to turn to when problems arose. I often saw how team members made the same mistakes and created workarounds individually to try to solve issues that, combined together, were a huge waste of time. This easily led to favoritism or comparisons among team members.

Are job descriptions easily accessible to everyone in the clinic? Everyone's job descriptions should be accessible to the whole clinic. If that's not possible, create a clinical operations guide that has job description information and is frequently updated as the operations in your clinic change or expand.

3. Identify your organization's structure.

What is your organization's structure? Who are your staff members, what do they do, and who do they report to? Who makes the decisions for which program? Does everyone know what this structure looks like? Again, this seems obvious, but I have found many organizations do not have this in place. I have seen employees fly under the radar when feedback never reaches supervisors and as such, employees never receive proper retraining. I have seen problems persist when individuals have no idea how to get proposed solutions in the hands of the decision-makers for the organization. It's a simple exercise that can help solidify the channels of communication.

During a team-bonding series with a group of residents, Lee asked them to create a visual representation of their organization's structure. The team had never been asked to do it before. The result was two white boards filled with a flow chart that would put a family tree to shame. Once it was in front of everyone, in addition to seeing how vast the network was, the residents had a much better grip on who to go to with specific questions and/or issues. The exercise took 30 minutes and may benefit residents within that organization for years to come.

CREATE A TEAM CULTURE

4. Define lines of communication.

Communication may seem intuitive, but it is not. Because of personality differences, you have to set rules for engagement. Define customs and courtesies early on. Everyone should address each other with respect.

Secondly, you need platforms to communicate information according to level of urgency. You can't communicate everything through email. Not all information needs to be given in a meeting that occupies time and keeps people from their primary duties. Prioritize what needs to be discussed in meetings and find more time-efficient ways for other information.

Daily huddles allow the dissemination of day-to-day information. For process improvement or discussion of systemic issues, a weekly or monthly meeting with all staff is more appropriate. For one-way communication, an email may suffice.

5. Delegate or leverage work.

Utilize your team. I cannot emphasize this enough. There is nothing worse than drowning in work while colleagues and technicians waste time on Facebook during the workday. This kills morale and is detrimental to team culture. There are ways to involve every team member.

Examine time allocation. Which team members have too much time, and who does not have enough? Tasks should be shared. Are there tasks right now that can be delegated to someone else who has more time? Delegate tasks and hold your team accountable. Require feedback and set that as the expectation.

Remember, these steps are just the starting point to creating an effective team.

STRATEGY AND TEAM BOND

Creating a true bond means creating a deeper purpose for the group that everyone can buy into.

Empowerment

Empower each member of the team. Do they have a role in the decision-making process? Does your decision-making process allow input from all levels of the organization?

Build and Maintain Camaraderie

Building camaraderie is not as difficult as you may think. You must show each member how their role in accomplishing the mission is vital and how roles overlap.

The phrase "not my job" is not allowed in our clinic. Instead, team members are encouraged to accomplish as much as they can within their scope of practice before handing it off to another team member.

Set Expectations

I cannot emphasize enough how important it is to lay out and identify expectations from the get-go. I would even argue that these expectations need to be outlined during the interview process. Expectations are the standard for yourself and others.

How do you address situations when team members do not meet expectations? Are feedback structures in place, including retraining when needed and defined disciplinary action when hard lines are crossed? Do team members find out they have made a mistake in a timely manner?

Trust and communication need to be the foundation for your team. If you cannot trust your team, or team members cannot com-

CREATE A TEAM CULTURE

municate with each other, problems will not get fixed in a timely manner, if at all.

On occasion, you may have to deal with inappropriate conversations. This is probably the hardest thing to address. This is typically a result of miscommunication or tension among staff. Gossip is inappropriate and more importantly, detrimental in the workplace. Make this known.

I consider gossip to be any conversation about a member of your team when you have no control or power to invoke change. This might mean one team member talking to a second about how a third team member made an error. Unless they are discussing how to help this team member, this is not productive and is detrimental to your environment and your team. If the team member who made the error is never informed, it is neither productive nor useful. In reality it's a disservice.

Changing Sentiments

Create an environment of safety. When people make mistakes, use it as a learning tool rather than berating them and threatening job termination. There's a great phrase we use in our house: "I never lose; I win or I learn."

Yes, certain lines cannot be crossed in medicine, especially in the realm of keeping our patients safe. But it is key to be transparent about your own mistakes and the lessons you've learned. You will be surprised how much this changes the dynamics of your team. This will pave the path toward process improvement and innovation instead of encouraging team members to hide mistakes or omit information for fear of termination. The more you can learn from each other's mistakes in a safe environment, the better and more efficient the environment will become.

Building Bridges

Building bridges means building a support system throughout your community. Your team is not just the people you work with. Other people also make the clinic run, such as IT, local pharmacies, and care management programs. Look outside of your defined area or clinic to create relationships with other organizations to take care of patients together.

Strategies and Schematics

Begin by creating checklists for your staff. This is a good way to create habits and ensure everything is completed in a systematic fashion. So much time can be wasted trying to reinvent a process a staff member is not familiar with.

Plans and strategies should be written down, but they're often not. Your checklists should outline specific roles and how the role fits in the larger scheme of things. Checklists are guidelines for all. While we should encourage following these guidelines on a daily basis, there will be times where the checklist may not be appropriate. When this occurs, does your team have the wherewithal to ask the right questions?

When learning how to approach medicine, I was constantly told, "Learn what is normal and you will never miss something abnormal." This is how I feel about strategies and checklists. Everyone should know what the normal operations look like. When changes have to be made to accommodate a new situation, like a COVID-19 pandemic, it is easier to create new processes when everyone understands what typical operations look like.

Make sure all the jobs in the clinic are assigned to someone.

CREATE A TEAM CULTURE

As physicians, we can't continue to put more tasks on ourselves with the attitude of "just get it done." Assign each task to someone on your team.

I emphasize assigning all tasks to a specific person for two reasons:

1. This helps to verify that people know how to do their job confidently. It creates continuity and stability.

2. Most importantly, it ensures that new jobs or tasks get incorporated into the day-to-day operations. Unexpected tasks or jobs cause a significant amount of distress to individuals and are a large contributor to burnout. If additional tasks are not accounted for, team members are likely sacrificing time from other aspects of their lives to complete these.

END GOAL: AN ACCOUNTABLE CLINIC

Above all, the purpose of creating a bonded team is so you all can utilize each other to achieve results. **This includes you as a person and physician.** There is nothing worse than drowning in work while colleagues or technicians use their time to shop online or are on social media for affairs not related to work. You can change your team culture. There are ways to involve every team member toward accomplishing a common goal. Set expectations early. Delegate tasks and hold others accountable. Inspire feedback and set realistic expectations.

As physicians, when we see a problem, our tendency is to take it on and fix it. There is a perception that we are solely responsible for the patients, a view that is reinforced by the current litigation and malpractice proceedings. But this responsibility and work needs to be shared with others. You must share it to create an environment where all the staff have the primary mission in sight and can take a more active role in everyday processes. Ultimately, this leads to better care of the patient. The patient can access a team that addresses their questions. Without that team approach, patients simply encounter a bottleneck while they wait for you, the provider, to call back and address all their questions.

It is also okay to create some duplication of roles. Encourage your team to have a primary and backup person for all positions. I'm a firm believer that responsibilities are carried out by individuals but should be assigned to a position. This may seem confusing initially, but we run into these issues when someone calls out sick (or for any other reason) or leaves a position. The work still needs to be done.

Lastly, continue to engage patients to be involved in their own care and in the administrative processes. I believe it is our obligation to help patients navigate this complex medical system. Ultimately, the patients are the consumers of this product that is medicine. This is a reality of American medicine. Sheltering patients from the difficulties in medicine prevents them from taking action against some of these injustices. Be transparent about what is going on.

Building a Team

Building a team does not have to be an arduous task. Instead, begin with commonality and purpose. To start, everyone on a team, no matter what their role is, should have an understanding of what the clinic's common purpose is. This can be done through training focused on creating common purpose charts, starting with whoever is in charge. Write a vision—what the clinic strives for under the leadership of that person as long as they are in charge. It should be clear, consistent, and reviewed every year and updated as needed.

CREATE A TEAM CULTURE

A strong starting point for a vision would be "to create a medical environment where patients, physicians, and everyone in between are working together toward better health."

The next step is to write a mission statement for the next three to five years. What are you trying to accomplish? If I was in a struggling clinic, the mission might be "to provide the best patient care possible while turning the clinic around."

After you've defined the vision and mission, write the objectives—how will you, as a team, accomplish the mission? What does the front desk need to do to improve the patient experience? How can team members help lighten the physicians' workloads so they can focus on their most important work? Write these objectives (usually five to 10) in clear terms.

Example objectives to accomplish your vision and mission might be these:

- Better patient care

- Good communication

- Preparedness

- Medical practice

- Accountability to your role

- Accountability to each other

Finally, we outline tactics—how you're going to achieve the objectives. If the objective is better patient care, one of the tactics to accomplish this might be saying "Hello" every time a patient walks in. These tactics outline the concrete actions the team can do right now. Each objective should have as many tactics as needed, as long as they all work toward accomplishing the mission and vision.

Once all of these items are completed, you will have completed a common purpose chart.

These charts should be created at virtually every level of your organization, from the top down. Once a common purpose has been defined by the person in the highest leadership role, the next person in the chain of command does the same thing. Everything on their common purpose chart must accomplish the vision, mission, objectives, and tactics of the common purpose chart before them. You can break these down all the way to the janitorial staff. Everyone's purpose must align with the purpose of the team.

This exercise helps to create a clear pathway for work to be accomplished as a team. Instead of unhealthy competition and finger-pointing between factions, groups in this environment will share resources while serving to accomplish the unified vision(s). It encourages support between groups and creates an understanding: "If we don't accomplish the overall goals together, we're not really accomplishing anything as a clinic."

Working in teams can be extremely difficult for physicians. After all, it is not typically part of our culture and training. When compared to business training, most physicians do not work in interdisciplinary teams during medical school and have very limited experience with teamwork during residency.

You can also use team-building exercises to foster a better sense of community among your team members. There are thousands of examples online.

Breaking Down Silos

For many of us, especially physicians early in our careers, there is very little or no time set aside for collaboration with other physicians and team members. I remember my early days as a new attending—it was a sprint into chaos with almost every minute of my

CREATE A TEAM CULTURE

day full of tasks and busywork. However, only through collaboration can we see innovation and create an opportunity to transform medicine. So how can we begin to incorporate this philosophy into our day-to-day?

Right now, many of you most likely see patients four to five days a week, and every minute is accounted for. This can be particularly true for employed physicians. A schedule packed with patients and inefficiencies will not allow space for collaboration with other physicians, administrators, or your team. When we think about why healthcare is not as innovative as it can be, this is why. Many of our primary care offices still struggle to bring their information and platforms online. We have not embraced what technology can do for us in changing the way we deliver medical care.

The medical field is severely siloed, even in our individual clinics.

Silos are enemies to teamwork.

This is what a silo looks like: the administrators are at the top, below them are the physicians and advanced practice practitioners, then nurses, techs, and front office staff. We all offer different perspectives and our missions are often interrelated and difficult to separate. How often do we all come together to make decisions that will impact the entire system? Commonly, our input is sought out in the last phase for final approval of a decision that was already made by administration. This is not collaboration.

We see this all too frequently: segregated groups convene in their own small groups—silos—where they commiserate with each other and work to achieve their own goals rather than the goals of the team as a whole. But as an organization, you can change this culture.

I have seen this done well. I have been part of organizations that expect their team members to collaborate with others both within and outside of their own organization. More importantly, they are given the time and platform to do so. While I was in the military, we had training days once a month where our entire medical group was closed to patient care for the purpose of training, troubleshooting, collaborating, and innovating. We discussed issues with the clinic, created action items, and assigned tasks. We created training platforms and ensured everyone was proficient in their roles. The regularly scheduled intervals allowed for follow-up and continued planning.

I have also seen well-intended efforts to start the collaboration process that lacked follow-through. The institutions I have been part of have attempted to facilitate collaborations, but they are typically in the form of a once-yearly faculty development or networking event. While great events, they require a large time commitment from all parties and at the end, what is the ultimate goal? After the event is over, we are still left with the same problem. No time was carved out of our schedules to take action. We had no flexibility to actively collaborate on projects or brainstorm new ideas based on what we discussed during the event. How fruitful are these events? For many of us, projects that will ultimately improve our work life are worked on after hours and on weekends. That is not sustainable and de-incentivizes individuals from taking on such roles.

Creating Stakeholder Teams for Collaboration

As we identify problems within our organizations, putting together teams with members who represent the various voices is paramount. This is how collaboration can start.

CREATE A TEAM CULTURE

We can start to facilitate a culture of collaboration within medicine. In our smaller organizations, this might begin by creating a monthly or every-other-month meeting with the key stakeholders either of the hospital, the clinic, or the surrounding resources to tackle these questions:

- What are our patients facing right now?
- How can we help each other out?
- Who is doing it right?

Then there's a crucial step: Organizations should create flexibility to allow key data sharing to occur during the business day.

Engaging Physicians for Problem-Solving Is Critical

For hospital systems and healthcare organizations, actively seeking the expertise of those who directly care for patients is paramount. Only by engaging them in the conversation can we create real solutions to the problems we face in medicine. These conversations will also facilitate system buy-in and implementation of new programs. This is where healthcare organizations recently have missed the mark.

As outlined by a 2017 *Harvard Business Review* article, physicians feel they have been left out of the collaborating team in key business and practice management decisions (van Biesen and Weisbrod, 2017). The competing agendas between business and clinical care as well as the lack of true collaboration is killing our field, costing our patients, and costing our profession. This is demonstrated by the numbers of physicians who leave medicine after they feel there is no other recourse.

STAY IN MEDICINE

For physicians and systems alike, it is crucial for physicians to become part of the decision-making structure.

Many physicians feel they are no longer part of the conversation, leading to increased resistance to company policies and decreased buy-in and innovation within organizations. **The truth is, when physicians are involved in administrative decisions, costs are reduced** (Sarto and Veronesi, 2016).

CREATE A TEAM CULTURE

TAKE 10

Quick exercise: Define the word *trust* without using the word in the definition.

It's not as easy as you'd think. In reality, we all have different definitions, depending on several different factors, including but not limited to upbringing, community, education, and experience.

Then, answer these questions to help you identify the path to an accountable clinic:

1. What is your clinic's mission? If you don't have one, set a group meeting time to develop one with your team.

2. Who are your team members and what are their roles?

3. Are your team members practicing at the top of their scope or ability?

4. What is their role in completing your clinic's mission?

CHAPTER 6 WRAP-UP

Because how you interact with your team is under your control, you can change your day-to-day experience for the better. Build a team with a common purpose whose mission is to provide better patient care, improve patient relationships, and run a smoothly operating, cost-efficient clinic. Connect with your team, build relationships with them, and establish trust. Then, as a group, evaluate each person's role and how they might be better utilized to distribute the administrative workload. Begin with the new standard of a daily team huddle to address problems and find solutions in a way that engages everyone.

Join the conversation at
StayInMedicine.com

7

Become a Physician Leader

> **Problem:** Medical school does not equip physicians with the leadership skills they need and are expected to have to run a clinic.
>
> **What you control:** Your efforts to continually become a better leader and enable others to lead.
>
> **Action item:** Take the time to learn leadership principles.

SEEK OUT LEADERSHIP TRAINING

Leadership skills, a necessity for physicians, weren't part of the curriculum when I was in medical school. And currently, a leadership skill set is still seen as an extra, rather than an essential skill vital to practicing medicine. We all understand we must lead, but no one shows us how to lead or what leadership in medicine means.

In fact, I think the medical culture does the opposite. In many ways, you are taught to be a subordinate. You are told where to go, how to dress, how to speak, and how to memorize information and regurgitate it back on exams or when diagnosing patients. Where is the opportunity to lead a team, before you become an attending?

How about opportunities to analyze the environment and come up with a plan? Or the chance to figure out team dynamics, key roles in communication, and dissemination of information?

I was taught how to lead in the military. It started with officer training school and resumed after medical school during my residency training at Eglin Air Force Base. During officer training school, I was assigned to leadership roles. I was told, "You are a military officer first, then a doctor." And I was given feedback depending on how effective I was at accomplishing my mission and managing my team. I learned to bring people together, to find common ground, and listen to different perspectives.

During residency, leadership training was part of our curriculum. I was "volun-told" to take on various non-medical jobs. We were expected to mentor our airmen, teach, communicate, inform, collaborate, and resolve conflicts, among other responsibilities. Working in teams was commonplace and expected. I remember one of my attendings telling me, "Prepare yourself. Your first job out of residency will be a leadership job." He was spot on. That was the expectation in the military. And my colleagues helped me along the way.

In my first job out of residency, leadership was expected and dictated by rank. I was in charge of conducting huddles and training my technicians in conjunction with my medical duties. The culture of leading and being led was everywhere. It was no surprise, coming out of training, that I was placed in a leadership position—an element leader to start, then medical director. This is the culture in the military. With seniority and rank, you will be in a leadership position. That's how the military works when you are an officer.

Now, in my role as an attending, I explain this concept and the importance of leadership to the medical students I teach, and they are stunned. "I wouldn't even know where to start," they say.

I relay stories on how much my leadership training has helped me in the practice of medicine and how these skills are vital to pulling a clinic together and resolving conflicts with patients and staff, among others. Currently, leadership training is offered to those seeking management roles as an extra or additional accreditation that must be sought out. This approach ignores the fact that for physicians, leadership is needed in their day-to-day jobs, whether they're formally in management or not. Currently, there is no prospect in medical school to make this part of the medical curriculum.

Throughout medical school training, there is opportunity for students to put these skills to action in the form of organizing health fairs and student-run clinics. There are also chances to implement educational programs for patients and communities. These are places where medical students can learn to lead and manage a team. The opportunity is there, however the crucial step of teaching these vital skills is absent.

> *Leadership in medicine used to be the expectation, and it should still be.*

It is not something reserved for the few exceptional students who seek out leadership opportunities. In a cross-sectional study looking at the top 100 U.S. hospitals in 2009, data suggested physician-led hospitals perform better, with higher-quality care (Goodall, 2011). Similar results were seen when looking at large hospital systems led by physicians in 2015.

We all need to be leaders in our role as doctors. The patients expect it and we should expect it of ourselves. Learning leadership should not be considered above and beyond the academic coursework. It needs to be taught. It needs to be ingrained in medical school just like it is ingrained in the military. Many organizations fail to adapt to the need for physician leadership as a way of keeping physicians engaged in medicine.

CHANGE CAN START WITH US

Change starts with us—with physicians. For those of us who never received formal training in leadership, know that this is an additional skill, akin to learning antibiotic stewardship. You must seek information. Learning how to lead, when to take the lead, or when to lead from behind are skills essential for running an effective team and for any level of problem-solving.

I was fortunate enough to be part of an organization that understands leadership training starts at every level and is actively developed over time. At every point in my military career, I was challenged to take on projects and actively engage in problem-solving and quality-improvement endeavors. My airmen had the same expectation. As their careers advanced, they too were given projects and teams to manage. The avenues for dissemination of information were clearly defined and the use of these avenues was encouraged. As a physician, I participated in policy-making for our hospital and for our base.

Why is this not the expectation in hospitals or outpatient organizations? At what point did physicians get carved out of the decision-making process? Were we even part of it to begin with? I fear that without leadership training, physicians will not see that their roles in committees are vital in shaping how medicine is delivered. These leadership roles need to be part of our jobs. And time should be committed to our service in these roles.

Here are some things physicians have to offer in leadership positions:

1. **Insight:** We are the bridge between what the patients need and the medical system. Most patients do not understand what is going on in the medical world around them. I don't blame them—it is hard for even me to keep up, some days. We know the battles that need to be fought and the questions that need to be answered.

2. **Data analysis:** Who else can analyze data like we can? Perhaps statisticians. But we have context. We analyze medical articles every day and break down that data in language patients are able to understand.

3. **Resiliency:** As physicians, we are the most resilient set of professionals I know. We are good at problem-solving, but we need dedicated time and space for that type of thinking, outside of patient care.

I have learned through leadership that when others make the rules without the contribution of those who do the work, everyone suffers.

> *Physicians need to be leaders in medicine, and leadership skills must be woven into our training.*

As a community, we need to change the way we think about leadership.

LEARNING LEADERSHIP

Leadership is a learned skill. No one is born with leadership skills, despite what people believe. Moreover, no one can ever perfect it—it's an evolving art. Like anything else, it takes study and practice. View it through the same lens as you approached medicine.

We've gone over many principles in this book for how to create a team. Start there. Until there are systems to incorporate leadership training into the standard medical school curriculum, we suggest this is a skill you actively seek. A lot of additional content is out there to help you. Take a formal course. There are online self-study courses or in-person classes. And for those of us who are busy moms or dads, there are always audiobooks and podcasts we can learn from during our commutes.

Seek mentorship from your leaders. Learn from those who have experience leading. This may require a change in attitude. As a medical student, I was afraid to ask my attending anything. I viewed it as a sign of weakness or a deficit of intelligence. So instead of asking, I would research everything on my own and waste a lot of time. If you see a great leader, approach them. If you're too shy, try following them on social media.

For those who are already in leadership positions, pave the way for others. Help create a curriculum or a pathway where this can be passed down to our future doctors. Encourage colleagues to enter leadership positions. Share your shortcomings in your own leadership.

Create a legacy of leadership.

Here are some basics to get you started:

Cultivate an environment of trust with your team and organization. Get to know your people and what motivates them. Knowing your people and what they are interested in can help improve your clinic and serve as professional development for your staff. If you know your MA wants to go to school to be a nurse, give them guidance.

Outline expectations. Expectations should be clear from all sides. Start with job descriptions. What do you expect from your colleagues? What do they expect from you? What do they expect from each other? Outlining this early will help prevent miscommunication among team members.

Empower team members. I learned the hard way that imposing process improvement directives on others without their input can backfire. As physicians, we know a lot, but we don't know it all. When there is a problem, I bring the problem first to the person who does the job. Their input is valuable and often their understanding of the job results in a solution that is more feasible and efficient for all.

Assess performance. Are the outcomes being measured in line with the expectations set forth by you and the organization? If expectations are not being met, how is feedback given? Is there a system in place to determine if this is a systemic issue, such as improper training, or an individual issue? When someone is not meeting expectations and others have to pick up the slack, it can lead to significant resentment and division of the team.

Clarify avenues of communication. How is information disseminated in your organization? If no infrastructure exists, this is where your leadership comes into play. You may have to assemble a team and create the avenues for communication.

Change the view on leadership. Yes, leadership comes with responsibility. I always remember the advice of a wise mentor: "Those who avoid leadership are subject to the decisions of others." Choosing a leadership position is choosing to stay part of the conversation that helps shape your environment.

TAKE 10

What leadership traits do you currently display in your day-to-day interactions with your team? Consider your performance in these areas (identify whether you do this, you don't do this, or you need to improve):

1. Relationships with team members: Do you know what's important to each person on your team, or something about what they are interested in?

2. Roles and responsibilities: When was the last time you looked at the job description for each member of your team? How do those descriptions translate into day-to-day expectations?

3. Clarify avenues of communication: What methods do you use to communicate with your team? Do you have a platform for team interaction on a regular basis (a team huddle, for example)? Are your methods effective?

4. Empowering your team: Do you show your team members that you value their expertise by asking for their input on task improvement efforts?

CHAPTER 7 WRAP-UP

Recognize that you can improve your day-to-day by taking on an active leadership role. As a physician, you are the leader of your patient-care team, but do you have the skills to lead effectively? Even though leadership skills weren't taught in medical school, they are crucial to aligning your team to effectively provide patient care and support you. Get to know your team members, discuss their roles and responsibilities with them, and engage them to perform at the top of their scope. Empower them to make decisions and handle some of the tasks that are weighing you down. Look for opportunities to grow your leadership skills because teamwork can calm some of the chaos you may be experiencing.

Join the conversation at
StayInMedicine.com

Change Can Start With You

I am just another physician looking for reasons to stay in medicine. I am wondering why my quandary to leave medicine is not about the patients. I love seeing patients. I love practicing medicine. Yet, like so many physicians, I am employed and wonder how we got where we are. Why do we have the perception that we have no voice and no power to protect ourselves or our patients from devastating systemic issues in healthcare today?

Healthcare needs to change, but you already know that. We are here to show you how **this change can start with you.** We must take the conversation a step further.

There's more to the problems the medical field is facing than we can solve individually in our everyday work environments. There are larger forces in motion, and we should attempt to look at the bigger picture.

When new physicians leave residency and begin their new jobs, they realize the challenges they face every day are not about practicing medicine. These challenges are about how we deliver care. We can lighten our day-to-day workload by engaging a true teamwork approach to patient care. For things to truly change, we must step back and look at medicine as a whole. We must become advocates.

Medicine as a business is growing, yet the paychecks received by those delivering care are not growing. Top executives from health insurance companies are making millions. But the patients are not any healthier, and they're paying more than they did 10 years ago for their healthcare. Who holds this system and its individuals accountable?

Physicians and healthcare providers need to continue to put the patient as first priority in all discussions surrounding healthcare and be an advocate for the patient when this does not occur.

We must continue to talk about issues and take it a step further to organize our resources for effective resolutions. There have been instances in the past when physicians and healthcare providers banded together to fight an issue and brought about powerful change. We need to continue making an effort. We see all the systemic issues, but we're not fighting them. To create change, we must organize. There's strength in numbers.

Physicians organizing can make a difference. It's worth sacrificing some of our time. Our communities need our expertise.

Healthcare providers have taken a stand against the NRA to advocate for gun regulation because we treat patients who suffer the consequences of gun violence. It has allowed us to study gun violence as the public health issue it is. It was a small win, because the U.S. still has a lot of gun violence, but now we're able to study it using government funds because physicians took a stand, banded together, and flooded social media. It was all over the news. There were pictures of surgeons' shoes covered in blood after trying to resuscitate a patient who had been shot.

This is an example of the power we have as providers and physicians. Similarly, residents have banded together to protest inhumane work environments by staging a walkout. We have more power than we think, especially when we work together for a cause.

We hope this book has helped you learn to create a team environment and improve your day-to-day operations. Beyond that, we encourage you to engage in matters outside your own clinic. As healthcare providers, we are in the best position to be advocates for our patients because we see both sides.

We can help patients understand the complexities of the healthcare system and prepare them to advocate for themselves while we continue to advocate for them. We are in the unique position to see how these system issues affect patients and the way we practice medicine.

Becoming an advocate is not just about changing the medical environment—it will help you reignite your passion for medicine. We got into medicine to help others. Whether it's becoming politically involved or just teaching others, physicians have to engage in more than just clinical care.

All this and more will be possible if we dare to start the conversation.

Engage your colleagues, read, get on social media, and engage your healthcare team and your patients. We are all stakeholders. We all have something to lose if we don't change the direction healthcare is headed for the better.

References

INTRODUCTION

Davenport, Liam. "'Alarming' Rate of Burnout in Med Students," Medscape, March 6, 2018. https://www.medscape.com/viewarticle/893466

McCarthy, Niall. "How U.S. Healthcare Spending Per Capita Compares With Other Countries," [Infographic] *Forbes*, August 8, 2019. https://www.forbes.com/sites/niallmccarthy/2019/08/08/how-us-healthcare-spending-per-capita-compares-with-other-countries-infographic/#7c3620fd575d

Pipes, Sally. "Government Policies Are Driving Doctors to Quit Health Care," *Forbes*, October 15, 2018. https://www.forbes.com/sites/sallypipes/2018/10/15/government-policies-are-driving-doctors-to-quit-health-care/?sh=44efd5ac2bf3

CHAPTER 1

Anderson, Pauline. "Physicians Experience Highest Suicide Rate of Any Profession," Medscape, 2018. https://www.medscape.com/viewarticle/896257

Farmer, Blake. "When Doctors Struggle With Suicide, Their Profession Often Fails Them," NPR, 2018. https://www.npr.org/sections/health-shots/2018/07/31/634217947/to-prevent-doctor-suicides-medical-industry-rethinks-how-doctors-work

Kane, Leslie, M.A. "Medscape Physician Compensation Report 2019," Medscape, 2019. https://www.medscape.com/slideshow/2019-compensation-overview-6011286 (requires free membership to access)

Kane, Leslie, M.A. "Medscape National Physician Burnout, Depression & Suicide Report 2019," Medscape, 2019. https://www.medscape.com/slideshow/2019-lifestyle-burnout-depression-6011056 (requires free membership to access)

Khullar, Dhruv. "Do You Trust the Medical Profession?" *The New York Times*, January 23, 2018. https://www.nytimes.com/2018/01/23/upshot/do-you-trust-the-medical-profession.html

Spector, Nicole. "The doctor is out? Why physicians are leaving their practices to pursue other careers," NBC News, 2018. https://www.nbcnews.com/business/business-news/doctor-out-why-physicians-are-leaving-their-practices-pursue-other-n900921

CHAPTER 2

Yarnall, M.D., Kimberly S. H.; Kathryn I. Pollak, Ph.D.; Truls Østbye, M.D., Ph.D.; Katrina M. Krause, M.A.; and J. Lloyd Michener, M.D. "Primary Care: Is There Enough Time for Prevention?" *Am. J. Public Health,* April 2003; 93(4): 635–641. doi: 10.2105/ajph.93.4.635; https://www.ncbi.nlm.nih.gov/pmc/articles/PMC1447803/

CHAPTER 3

Sinsky, M.D., Christine; Lacey Colligan, M.D.; Ling Li, Ph.D.; Mirela Prgomet, Ph.D.; Sam Reynolds, MBA; Lindsey Goeders,

REFERENCES

MBA; Johanna Westbrook, Ph.D.; Michael Tutty, Ph.D.; and George Blike, M.D. "Allocation of Physician Time in Ambulatory Practice: A Time and Motion Study in 4 Specialties," *Annals of Internal Medicine*, September 6, 2016. https://www.acpjournals.org/doi/10.7326/M16-0961?url_ver=Z39.88-2003&rfr_id=ori:rid:crossref.org&rfr_dat=cr_pub%20%200pubmed

Overhage, M.D., Ph.D., J. Marc; David McCallie Jr., M.D. "Physician Time Spent Using the Electronic Health Record During Outpatient Encounters: A Descriptive Study," *Annals of Internal Medicine*, January 14, 2020. https://pubmed.ncbi.nlm.nih.gov/31931523/

CHAPTER 4

Herrera, Tim. "A Deceptively Simple Way to Find More Happiness at Work," *The New York Times*, April 7, 2019. https://www.nytimes.com/2019/04/07/smarter-living/how-to-be-happier-at-work.html

45 CFR Parts 147 and 158, *Federal Register*, Vol. 84, No. 229, Wednesday, November 27, 2019, Proposed Rules: "Transparency in Coverage," File code CMS–9915–P, RIN 0938–AU04. Executive Order on Improving Price and Quality Transparency in American Healthcare to Put Patients First. https://www.govinfo.gov/content/pkg/FR-2019-11-27/pdf/2019-25011.pdf

CHAPTER 5

Masters, M.D., Philip A. "The isolation and loneliness that physicians experience," *KevinMD.com*, May 7, 2019. https://www.kevinmd.com/blog/2019/05/the-isolation-and-loneliness-that-physicians-experience.html

Pearl, M.D., Robert. "Physician Burnout: Isolation, Loneliness and the Loss of the American Hospital," *Forbes*, August 12, 2019. https://www.forbes.com/sites/robertpearl/2019/08/12/physician-burnout-isolation/#39476c7b58a0

Rubin, M.D., MBA, CPHQ, Richard. "Physician Burnout and the Loss of Collegial Relationships: A Reversible Trend?" StuderGroup.com, February 8, 2016. https://www.studergroup.com/resources/articles-and-industry-updates/insights/february-2016/physician-burnout-and-the-loss-of-collegial-relati

Shanafelt, M.D., Tait D.; Colin P. West, M.D., Ph.D.; Christine Sinsky, M.D.; Daniel V. Satele, B.S.; Lindsey E. Carlasare, MBA; Lotte N. Dyrbye, M.D., MHPE. "Changes in Burnout and Satisfaction With Work-Life Integration in Physicians and the General US Working Population Between 2011 and 2017," *Mayo Clinic Proceedings*, 2019; 94(9): 1681–1694. https://www.mayoclinicproceedings.org/article/S0025-6196(18)30938-8/fulltext

West, M.D., Ph.D., Colin P., Liselotte N. Dyrbye, M.D., MHPE; Jeff T. Rabatin, M.D., M.Sc.; et al. "Intervention to Promote Physician Well-being, Job Satisfaction, and Professionalism: A Randomized Clinical Trial," *JAMA Intern Med.*, 2014; 174(4):527–533. doi:10.1001/jamainternmed.2013.14387; https://jamanetwork.com/journals/jamainternalmedicine/fullarticle/1828744

CHAPTER 6

Sarto, F. and G. Veronesi. "Clinical leadership and hospital performance: assessing the evidence base," *BMC Health Serv Res.*, 2016; 16(Suppl 2): 169. Published online May 24, 2016. doi: 10.1186/s12913-016-1395-5; https://www.ncbi.nlm.nih.gov/pmc/articles/PMC4896259/

Van Biesen, Tim, and Josh Weisbrod. "Doctors Feel Excluded from Health Care Value Efforts," *Harvard Business Review*, October 6, 2017. https://hbr.org/2017/10/doctors-feel-excluded-from-health-care-value-efforts

REFERENCES

CHAPTER 7

Goodall, Amanda H. "Physician-leaders and hospital performance: Is there an association?" *Social Science & Medicine*, August 2011; 73(4): 535–539. https://doi.org/10.1016/j.socscimed.2011.06.025; https://www.sciencedirect.com/science/article/abs/pii/S0277953611003819

Acknowledgments

I want to thank my family for the endless support with a reach so vast, it followed me literally around the world.

First, to my husband, my life companion . . . we started this adventure as kids. You didn't know what you were getting into, but you took the leap anyway despite our different ethnicities, religions, political ideologies, social economic backgrounds . . . come to think of it, just about everything about us is different. Nine moves later, among four states and a short jump across the "Pond," you are still by my side and down for whatever comes. Despite all our differences, our core is the same and we push each other to become the best versions of ourselves. We are an example of what a partnership can look like. I thank you most of all for caring for me when I was too busy taking care of others to bother taking care of myself.

To Logan and Alina—you both remind me every day what this is all about. Those precious moments keep me going and remind me why it is so important. Logan—you are a healer in the making. You have a way of reading emotion in others and curing bad days with laughter. Alina, you are fierce and headstrong—I don't wonder where you have gotten it from because I know exactly where. Never lose it.

To my family, we are a village in all senses of the word—a place for respite, support, and rejuvenation.

Queridos Madre y Padre, gracias por enseñarme la importancia de una vida de servicio. Siempre defendían a los demás, y eran un refugio para aquellos en necesidad. Trataban a todos como familia. Sin importar las circunstancias complicadas de la vida, para ustedes era simple, tratar al prójimo como un ser humano y cuidarnos unos a los otros. Sin importar lo poco que tenían, siempre encontraban para los demás. Nunca se daban por vencidos a los retos de la vida. Incluso cuando estoy al borde de rendirme, escucho aquella frase que solían repetir, <<todo tiene remedio>>, y me hace seguir adelante.

To my siblings: Jose, Julio, Juan Luis, Luis, and Angela—we are a force, the original and unbeknownst team. The amount of support I have received from all of you over the years has made my journey possible. Chelo, the number of times you fixed my POS car so I could get to college. Julio, being in the stands supporting me in sports when our parents couldn't. Luis, always being the "realist" and lending a rational solution to any problem. Angie, being the voice of reason, perpetual cheerleader, and accountability partner in all I do. There is nothing we haven't been able to figure out. No matter where we are in life, our ability to band together, support, and carry each other is *the* true gift.

My extended village: Collette—What can I say, my sister from another mother and father? No matter where we are in the world, we can always pick up where we left off like no time has gone by. You, better than most, understand why we push forward. We started as two poor kids trying to find a way into medicine. Fast-forward 18 years, and we propel our careers keeping those two young girls at heart.

ACKNOWLEDGMENTS

Gina, an earnest, caring, and compassionate soul. You always find a solution even when it seems impossible. I have learned to be a better mother because of you. It is a true honor to call you a friend.

The "tribunal," our beloved nickname for the fearless three—Ms. Marie Washington, Ms. Donna Lorenzo, and Ms. Serena Smith. Your selfless commitment to bring diversity into medicine is inspirational. I beat the statistics because of you three.

Physician Moms Group (PMG)—You have given a voice to female physicians and a professional network unrivaled in my professional experience thus far. Unknowingly, you were there for me and my family when we were trying to rebuild after Hurricane Maria. You embody the best of our profession: banding together and supporting and lifting each other. I look forward to meeting many of you in the future and hope this book helps others as this group has helped me.

To our military family scattered all over the world; Amanda and Jin O., thank you for showing us the ropes in a foreign land when Lee and I were just starting our family and knew no one. You are the best the military has to offer. Most of all, thank you for lending your couch when I was just too exhausted to drive all the way home. Jin, thank you for carrying me forward when I thought I could no longer, showing me trash-talking PT sessions are better than any other therapy. P.S., I still hold the fastest Nexplanon removal record.

Dr. Scheivenin, Dr. Dooley, Dr. Persons—thank you for pushing me into leadership and showing me the value of my voice. I never saw myself as a leader but remembered all of your discussions, stepping up to meet the challenge because it was needed, not necessarily because I wanted to. You exemplify integrity in medicine and I hope I can exemplify the same.

STAY IN MEDICINE

Jessica Lotridge, Jaydee Lumbad, Tina Nguyen, Danielle Dufresne—one of the most underestimated parts of any journey is knowing that you are not going through it alone. I am thankful to have experienced this adventure with such amazing female leaders, physicians, and friends.

RAF Lakenheath FM Blue Team—the team that I'm constantly trying to recreate everywhere I go. Amaya, Auld, Belise, Taylor, Jauch—I learned teamwork and camaraderie through you and the biggest lesson of all: when you invest in each other, everyone wins. Thank you for taking Logan with no notice at 2 a.m. when I was called into the hospital, for never backing down from a challenge at work, and for bringing laughter into the workplace. Thank you for trusting me with yours when it was your turn to go.

Drexel Family Medicine—to my colleagues and residents. I thought I knew resiliency before arriving here, but I was greatly mistaken. What a ride. Despite the walls collapsing we find a way to band together to keep them up so we can survive and thrive. It has been truly amazing working alongside all of you. I have found so many mentors and grown in ways I did not know was possible. Working with you has allowed me clarity of purpose and resolve. We do this because we care, we work for each other, and we make sure we pass on a legacy that others can be proud of and remember.

To the Aloha Publishing team—thank you for your enduring patience, guidance, and mentorship with this process. I never thought I would be an author, but with your powers of persuasion and support, I am thankful we are able to bring this message to individuals struggling to stay in medicine. I'd like to thank my family, extended family, education, friends, colleagues, and Maryanna Young, Megan Terry, Jennifer Regner, and the rest of the team at Aloha Publishing for helping this book come to life.

About the Authors

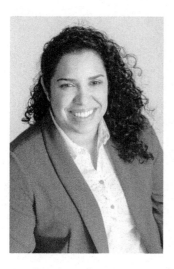

JANET CRUZ, M.D.

Dr. Janet Cruz is a board-certified family medicine physician in Philadelphia, Pennsylvania. She was born in Morristown, New Jersey, to Puerto Rican parents. She received her undergraduate degree in biology from Montclair State University, where she also served as an EMT. She attended medical school at the University of Medicine and Dentistry of New Jersey–New Jersey Medical School (UMDNJ), where she enjoyed and learned to care for patients in urban settings and communities.

She completed residency training and worked as Chief Resident at Eglin Air Force Base Family Medicine Program in Northwest Florida. Dr. Cruz served as a United States Air Force military physician at RAF Lakenheath Air Base in the United Kingdom and Dover Air Force Base in Delaware, where in addition to her clinical responsibilities, she coordinated training programs for wartime contingencies, humanitarian assistance, and disaster relief response.

With a particular interest in women's health, sexual health, and adolescent and college medicine, she currently works in an academic setting, completing work as a medical director to an outpatient clinic and as an inpatient attending while teaching medical students and family medicine residents. In 2020, Dr. Cruz served on the front lines of the public health response to the COVID-19 pandemic in Philadelphia.

She currently resides in the Philadelphia, Pennsylvania, suburbs with her husband, Lee, and their two children, Logan and Alina.

Awards and Honors

- Residency Teaching Award (2019)
- Meritorious Service Medal (2016)
- Air Force Achievement Medal (2015)
- Company Grade Office of the Quarter, 48th Medical Operations Squadron, RAF Lakenheath, United Kingdom (2014)
- Meritorious Unit Award (2014)
- Resident Mentor Award, Eglin Air Force Base Family Medicine Residency, 98th Medical Group, Eglin Air Force Base (2013)
- Air Force Longevity Service (2013)
- Air Force Overseas Ribbon Long (2013)
- Resident of the Year, Eglin Air Force Hospital, 98th Medical Group, Eglin Air Force Base (2012-2013)

ABOUT THE AUTHORS

- National Defense Service Medal (2012)
- Global War on Terrorism Service Medal (2011)
- Nuclear Deterrence Operations Service Medal (2012)
- 1st Year Excellence in Obstetrics Award, 98th Surgical Squadron, Eglin Air Force Hospital, 98th Medical Group, Eglin Air Force Base (2010-2011)
- Internal Medicine, Outstanding Service Intern of the Year, Eglin Air Force (2010-2011)
- Air Force Training Ribbon (2010)

STAY IN MEDICINE

LEE M.J. ELIAS

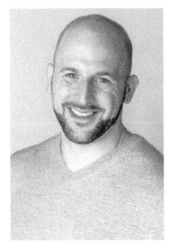

Lee Elias's credentials are rooted in sports, marketing, and management. He is a graduate of Montclair State University in Upper Montclair, New Jersey, with a B.A. in broadcasting and an M.S. degree in sports management from Drexel University in Philadelphia, Pennsylvania.

Lee is the founder of Game Seven Group, an organization that works with leaders to help them unlock excellence, reach their potential, and ultimately win using the spirit and culture of a professional sports organization. He is also the co-founder of Hockey Wraparound, Sports Achievements, and Ultimate Sports Nation, all of which are companies that work to make the game of hockey more enjoyable and accessible to the world.

Lee is also a professional speaker and team-bonding coach for various organizations in the business, nonprofit, medical, and sports worlds. He is the host of the WeLive.Hockey Podcast, Our Kids Play Hockey and co-host of Geeks Who Like Sports, all which can be found on all major podcast providers.

He served as a coach full time in 2007, at the age of 22, when he was named the general manager and head coach of the Montclair State University Ice Hockey team. During his time with the program, the team saw a dramatic rise from the bottom of the league to annually competing for both regional and national ranking.

In 2015, Lee was named a member of the coaching staff to the Peterborough Phantoms of the English Premier Ice Hockey League (EPIHL). In his first year with the organization, the team made

ABOUT THE AUTHORS

a dramatic turnaround from being near the bottom of the league during the prior year to winning the league's playoff championship. In addition to coaching, Lee also served as a member of the organization's media team.

Lee's other sports work experiences include serving the National Hockey League as the Coordinator of the NHL Network during its first season in the USA and working as a camera director for the New York Rangers and New York Knicks at Madison Square Garden. Beyond that, he served as a production specialist with the Pensacola Blue Wahoos (Cincinnati Reds AA) during their inaugural season.

In addition to his sports experience, in 2010 Lee was hired by LocalEdge, a Division of Hearst Media Services. With the company, he helped small-to-medium-sized businesses create digital plans focusing on search engine optimization, search engine marketing, social media marketing, and mobile marketing, among other solutions. Lee also was responsible for development of new consultants and assisting with product development, marketing, product expertise, and public speaking.

Lee is the award-winning author of *Think Like a Fan: Invest in Your Fans So They Invest in You*; *Win: What Every Team Needs to Know to Create a Championship Culture*; and co-author of *Stay in Medicine*. He was named to Drexel's 40 under 40 class of 2018.

He currently resides in the Philadelphia, Pennsylvania, suburbs with his wife, Janet, and their two children, Logan and Alina.

Join Our Community

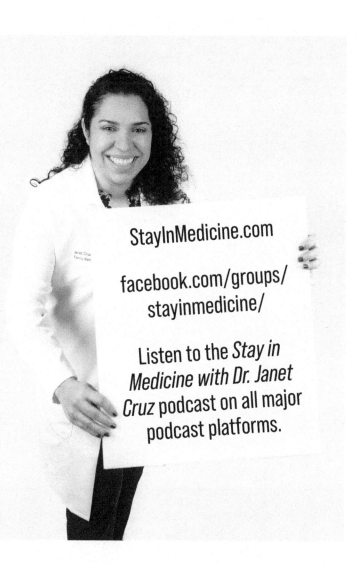

AlohaPublishing.com

Made in the USA
Coppell, TX
28 April 2021